T0186687

"This very engaging book, written by a high functioning survivor of a traumatic brain injury, gives an introspective and critical account of what it actually feels like to suffer a brain injury and 'come through the other side.' Christopher Yeoh integrates his phenomenological experience of brain injury with science, literature, autobiography, and philosophy, resulting in an extremely readable account of his experience. It provides a real 'insider's view' of brain injury not possible to capture in a purely academic textbook. For this reason, the book will be of huge importance not only to the individuals and their families affected by brain injury, but also the clinicians involved in their care and rehabilitation."

– Rudi Coetzer, Consultant Neuropsychologist,
North Wales Brain Injury Service, Betsi Cadwaladr UHB NHS Wales
and Senior Lecturer in Clinical Neuropsychology,
School of Psychology, Bangor University, UK

"Christopher's poignant narrative of his recovery and rehabilitation shows how personal characteristics and social resources interact to overcome the serious aftermath of severe traumatic brain injury. This is a balanced and insightful account of loss, challenge and triumph. He writes with humility and humour, whilst never masking the devastation the injury caused for him and his loved ones. Many inspiring books are written by survivors; *A Different Perspective After Brain Injury* will strike a chord with people grappling with changes to self in the context of any major life change. This is also an invaluable resource for clinicians, researchers and educators who seek a deeper understanding of the experience of brain injury."

– Professor Tamara Ownsworth, School of Applied Psychology,
Griffith University, Australia

A Different Perspective After Brain Injury

While preparing for his travel adventures into a world he had yet to explore, Christopher Yeoh was involved in a road traffic accident and experienced something few others would be "privileged" to witness: eight days in a coma, more than a year in and out of hospital and a gradual reintroduction to the world of work.

A Different Perspective After Brain Injury: A Tilted Point of View is written entirely by the survivor, providing an unusually introspective and critical personal account of life following a serious blow to the head. It charts the initial insult, early rehabilitation, the development of understanding, the return of emotion, both moments of triumph and regression into depression, the exercise of reframing how a brain injury is perceived and the return to work. It also describes the mental adjustments of awareness and acceptance alongside the physical recovery process.

Readily accessible to the general public, this book will also be of particular interest to professionals involved in the care of those who have incurred significant brain injuries, brain injury survivors, their families and friends, and also those who fund and organise health and social care. It is hoped that the author's account will provide a degree of understanding of what living with a hidden disability is really like.

Christopher Yeoh is a holder of an LLB and LLM from the London School of Economics and practises securities law as a solicitor of England and Wales at a major global law firm. After his adventure he now runs a multi-award-winning food and travel blog at quieteating.com and is a featured photographer in the *Telegraph* and *Sunday Times* newspapers.

Life after brain injury is not something less – just something different.

After Brain Injury: Survivor Stories
Series Editor: Barbara A. Wilson

This new series of books is aimed at those who have suffered a brain injury and their families and carers. Each book focuses on a different condition, such as face blindness, amnesia and neglect, or diagnosis, such as encephalitis and locked-in syndrome, resulting from brain injury. Readers will learn about life before the brain injury, the early days of diagnosis, the effects of the brain injury, the process of rehabilitation and life now. Alongside this personal perspective, professional commentary is also provided by a specialist in neuropsychological rehabilitation, making the books relevant for professionals working in rehabilitation such as psychologists, speech and language therapists, occupational therapists, social workers and rehabilitation doctors. They will also appeal to clinical psychology trainees and undergraduate and graduate students in neuropsychology, rehabilitation science and related courses who value the case study approach.

With this series, we also hope to help expand awareness of brain injury and its consequences. The World Health Organisation has recently acknowledged the need to raise the profile of mental health issues (with the WHO Mental Health Action Plan 2013–20) and we believe there needs to be a similar focus on psychological, neurological and behavioural issues caused by brain disorder, and a deeper understanding of the importance of rehabilitation support. Giving a voice to these survivors of brain injury is a step in the right direction.

Published titles:

Surviving Brain Damage After Assault
From Vegetative State to Meaningful Life
By Barbara A. Wilson, Samira Kashinath Dhamapurkar, and Anita Rose

Life After Encephalitis
A Narrative Approach
By Ava Easton

A Different Perspective After Brain Injury
A Tilted Point of View
By Christopher Yeoh

A Different Perspective After Brain Injury

A Tilted Point of View

Christopher Yeoh

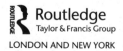
LONDON AND NEW YORK

First published 2018
by Routledge
2 Park Square, Milton Park, Abingdon, Oxon OX14 4RN

and by Routledge
711 Third Avenue, New York, NY 10017

Routledge is an imprint of the Taylor & Francis Group, an informa business

© 2018 Christopher Yeoh

The right of Christopher Yeoh to be identified as author of this work has been asserted by him in accordance with sections 77 and 78 of the Copyright, Designs and Patents Act 1988.

All rights reserved. No part of this book may be reprinted or reproduced or utilised in any form or by any electronic, mechanical, or other means, now known or hereafter invented, including photocopying and recording, or in any information storage or retrieval system, without permission in writing from the publishers.

Trademark notice: Product or corporate names may be trademarks or registered trademarks, and are used only for identification and explanation without intent to infringe.

British Library Cataloguing in Publication Data
A catalogue record for this book is available from the British Library

Library of Congress Cataloging in Publication Data
Names: Yeoh, Christopher, author.
Title: A different perspective after brain injury: a tilted point of view / Christopher Yeoh.
Description: Milton Park, Abingdon, Oxon; New York, NY: Routledge, 2018. | Series: After brain injury: survivor stories | Includes bibliographical references and index.
Identifiers: LCCN 2017004554 | ISBN 9781138055643 (hbk : alk. paper) | ISBN 9781138055650 (pbk : alk. paper) | ISBN 9781315165783 (ebk)
Subjects: LCSH: Yeoh, Christopher–Health. | Brain damage–Patients–Rehabilitation–Biography. | Head–Wounds and injuries–Patients–Biography. | People with disabilities–Biography. | Chronically ill–Social conditions.
Classification: LCC RC387.5 .Y46 2018 | DDC 617.4/81044092 [B] –dc23
LC record available at https://lccn.loc.gov/2017004554

ISBN: 978-1-138-05564-3 (hbk)
ISBN: 978-1-138-05565-0 (pbk)
ISBN: 978-1-315-16578-3 (ebk)

Typeset in Times New Roman
by Deanta Global Publishing Services, Chennai, India

For those without voices, my fellow traumatic brain injury survivors and their families.

Never lose hope.

Contents

Foreword

I first met Christopher when he was transferred from hospital in France to the Wellington Hospital in London, nearly three weeks after he had sustained multiple injuries, including a very severe traumatic brain injury, in a cycling accident.

At that time, as a result of the brain injury, he was confused and did not know where he was or the date. He tended to get agitated on the ward, he had no insight into the fact that he was unable to stand without support, and thus needed a carer in his room at all times to prevent him getting out of bed and falling. He also needed tube-feeding, he was not yet continent, and he complained of double vision. His limbs, however, were strong.

One to two weeks later, about four weeks after the injury, he became able to remember the date and where he was; he became less agitated and an MRI head scan showed changes consistent with a severe (Grade III) traumatic axonal injury.

To a lay or uninformed reader, this medical information may seem at best irrelevant and at worst intrusive, and, for the neurologist, self-serving, emphasising the doctor's knowledge and the patient's current and future dependency, but this is not the intention. On the contrary, it is important to document the severity of the injury because this emphasises the remarkable nature of Christopher's rehabilitation. For the majority of people, with such insults to the brain and with "usual" care, their subsequent recovery would not be sufficient to enable a full-time return to their previous work.

The fact that this was possible in Christopher's case can be attributed to a number of factors. He was not disadvantaged before the injury, in fact, he clearly performed at an exceptional level in many areas, and he had not had previous psychological difficulties or problems with alcohol or drug misuse. He had considerable support from his family and (almost) seamless support, treatment and rehabilitation from the time of the accident until recently, three and a half years after the injury.

Christopher was thus able to confront, explore and gradually resolve many of the problems he met over the last three years, during his return to independence and then his return to work. He has been able to relearn how to coordinate not only his physical but also his mental and emotional functions, and to know and manage his "self." His journey is eloquently described in this book and symbolised by the circuit of Annapurna completed by Christopher and his father at the end of 2016.

Christopher takes us through his early inpatient rehabilitation and subsequent reacquisition of insight, understanding and emotions, to the extent that he can now write about the difficulties he has encountered informatively and with humour. He explains in this book how, with perseverance, difficulties which would otherwise be perceived as deficits can resolve into a positive awareness of change as a result of injury, an ability to "deal with conflict by facing the consequences of [his] decisions," and an ability to build hope for the future.

This is therefore a rare volume, a readable story about events over three and a half years after a severe traumatic brain injury, which emphasises the effectiveness of informed support, tailored rehabilitation, personal exploration and the development of optimism over an extended period of time. For so many people after a severe traumatic brain injury, the lack of ongoing support and treatment over several years post-injury results in progress being stalled by secondary depression, encountered by Christopher as "The Bleakness," and a failure to resolve the difficulties associated with change post-injury. This book, however, shows how it is possible to overcome such difficulties with the right support and with the persistence to regain confidence, hope and a good quality of life, demonstrating that every effort should be made to pursue this treatment model.

A Different Perspective After Brain Injury: A Tilted Point of View should therefore be read by every professional involved in the care of those who have had significant brain injuries, brain injury survivors, their families and friends, and also by those who fund and organise health and social care, many of whom often know little about the difficulties confronted by people for whom they provide care, particularly in the context of the "invisible" difficulties that follow traumatic brain injury.

– Dr Richard Greenwood, BA, MB, BChir, MD, FRCP
Consultant Neurologist
December 2016

Series foreword

After Brain Injury: Survivor Stories was launched in 2014 to meet the need for a series of books aimed at those who have suffered a brain injury and their families and carers. Brain disorders can be life-changing events with far-reaching consequences. However, in the current climate of cuts to funding and service provision for neuropsychological rehabilitation, there is a risk that people whose lives have been transformed by brain injury may be left feeling isolated with little support.

So many books on brain injury are written for academics and clinicians and filled with technical jargon, and so are of little help to those directly affected. Instead, this series offers a much-needed personal insight into the experience, as each book is written by a survivor, or group of survivors, who are living with the very real consequences of brain injury. Each book focuses on a different condition, such as face blindness, amnesia and neglect, or diagnosis, such as encephalitis and locked-in syndrome, resulting from brain injury. Readers will learn about life before the brain injury, the early days of diagnosis, the effects of the brain injury, the process of rehabilitation and life now.

Alongside this personal perspective, professional commentary is also provided by a specialist in neuropsychological rehabilitation. The historical context, neurological state of the art, and data on the condition, including the treatment, outcome and follow-up, will also make these books appealing to professionals working in rehabilitation, such as psychologists, speech and language therapists, occupational therapists, social workers and rehabilitation doctors. This series will also be of interest to clinical psychology trainees and undergraduate and graduate students in neuropsychology, rehabilitation science and related courses who value the case study approach as a complement to the more academic books on brain injury.

With this series, we also hope to help expand awareness of brain injury and its consequences. The World Health Organisation has recently acknowledged the need to raise the profile of mental health issues (with the WHO

Mental Health Action Plan 2013–20) and we believe there needs to be a similar focus on psychological, neurological and behavioural issues caused by brain disorder, and a deeper understanding of the importance of rehabilitation support. Giving a voice to these survivors of brain injury is a step in the right direction.

Prof. Barbara A. Wilson, OBE, PhD, DSc, CPsychol,
FBPsS, FmedSC, AcSS
Clinical Neuropsychologist
January 2017

Acknowledgements

I would like to thank the countless people that have helped me on my adventure. There are almost too many to recount, so apologies if I have missed anyone. I express my gratitude to the staff at St Claude, Jean Minjoz, Mile End, University College, Royal London and Wellington hospitals, the National Hospital of Neurology and Neuroscience, the Oliver Zangwill Centre, and Headway, the brain injury association.

I would also like to thank the following people in particular who helped me return to normal, as well as those that provided a helping hand by pointing out areas which might benefit from additional crafting in my story. These are the various doctors, therapists, colleagues and friends.

Richard Greenwood, Guillaume Besch, Tim Lloyd, Christopher Bentley, Douglas Harrison, Mark Harvey, Teresa Clark, Emma Wilson, Freya Bell, Darren Mockler, Dharsha Navaratnam, Emma Dawson, Bonnie-Kate Dewar, Anna Meadow, Mary Summers, Danielle Day, Dominique St Clair Miller, Tullia Buck, Trudi Edginton, Barbara Wilson, Jill Winegardner, Leyla Prince, Alison Lawrence, Jessica Fish, Amy Neeb, Kris Wong, Heyling Chan, Kenneth Yu, David Dunnigan, Stewart Dunlop, Julian Barrow, Richard Johnson, Yasuko Moriwaki, Eric Green, Ayan Koshal, Daisy Cheung, James Harmer, Julia Machin, Dorothy Bidmead, Lucy Kennedy, Anna Cuthbert and Joanna Saw.

Most of all I would like to thank my family who endured this rather traumatic, stressful and exhausting process – my father, my mother and my younger brother. Words cannot express the gratitude I feel. Brain injury is truly something that challenges family ties.

Preface

This book is about me, egotistical as that may sound. It is about one of those occasions when a person is finally getting used to the work treadmill but then promptly gets knocked off, in my case, literally. While on holiday pedalling around on my push-cycle, I was unwillingly and forcibly ejected. I then spent the next two years on a longer vacation than I hoped, in and out of hospital.

Once I was done with that, back in normal society with a bit more time to think, I became a bit fed up with constant repetitions of my character-building exercises. I thought that there must be a better way to relate my experiences of an interesting life. For a time I toyed with the idea of maybe carrying around a recorded monologue to play back or a little pamphlet to hand out when asked. However, this approach would unlikely endear me to others, so I shelved those ideas. I also noticed that the aftermath of head injury seemed sadly underexplored; the existing popular literature seemed to concentrate on the immediate treatment, not the years following the initial insult. In contrast, although the medical literature provided observations over a longer time frame, these consisted very much of notes by physicians about their patients and lacked a first-person perspective. It then struck me that there was a way to deal with all of these problems with one fell stroke: writing my story.

So here are my memoirs of my recovery distilled down into a more readable form. My autobiography begins with my touch-and-go days in hospital, progresses through my accelerated adolescence and consequential discharge from inpatient hospital life, advances to my outpatient treatment and rehabilitation, and concludes with my return to work and a fresh start. Interspersed with this chronological tale, I include my consideration of less tactile elements to provide a bit of a breather from my action-packed "adventure."

Through my account, the hope is that it will help people understand why brain injury survivors act in seemingly bizarre ways at times, why they seem so hopelessly lost, why they seem so bitterly angry and why they look so heartbreakingly sad. Yet if the only thing that you come away with after reading this book is a glimpse of what living with a traumatic brain injury is like, I will be wholly satisfied.

I hope you find reading my story interesting, enlightening and perhaps even enjoyable.

Christopher Yeoh, LLB, LLM
Solicitor of England and Wales
December 2016

The start of the (almost) end

What would you do to have your slate wiped clean? To be able to remake yourself as you wished? To have an opportunity to start anew? While staring one day in the mirror, I thought that there must be more to life than sitting and dreaming about adventures. Perhaps I could live them. Now that would be something worth writing about.

Thus began my adventure of a lifetime. Here I was, enjoying one of those iconic moments in life, having trekked the Inca trail and finally arrived at its end: Machu Picchu. The weather was a bit humid but enjoyably warm, a nice change from my accustomed climate in dreary, cold and wet London. As I climbed the steps to a higher elevation, the humidity dropped away, leaving me to bask in the glory of the sun. What better place to get a tan than Machu Picchu, the ancient city of the Incas at 2,400 metres above sea level, the home of the famous sun god worshippers? Arriving at the top almost made the physical torment and mental strain worthwhile.

While admiring the sights, I was dreaming about the things to come on this journey of a lifetime. In my time off I planned to move from trekking to the roof of the world to plumbing the depths of the sea by diving with the sharks in the Galapagos Islands. The adventure would not stop there as I would then enjoy the rather more sedate manner of the quiet giant turtles. This would be in contrast to "revelling in" the company of the infuriating mosquitoes in the Amazon rainforest.

Land-based mammals would not be ignored, as I would then embark on a trip to Botswana for a two-week safari to be within petting distance of the wildlife. I also planned to do more constructive things during this break, such as learning how to dive, drive and jump from a plane, all the requisite elements of a modern man of adventure. At times, I had to try and suppress the inclination to jump for joy. I had so much to look forward to.

I am getting a bit ahead of myself here and some introductions are in order. I wish I could start with a pithy one-liner, but I think the best way of describing me would be as an orphan of the world; I had lived in so many places and could not readily call any one place my home. I also worked as a lawyer, a much-discussed profession. There are reasons why there are so many TV dramas about being a lawyer; it seems to be a life full of thrills and daily excitement. There never seems to be a dull moment on the silver screen. Although the truth is that when you are finally practising, the daily trudge is rather less dramatic.

Here I have a confession to make. My opening, extolling the virtues of the Inca trail, is all a fabrication. As people sometimes complain, I have a vivid imagination. Machu Picchu was where I was supposed to be, but I missed out. Unexpectedly, I would spend my time off in the most expensive of places: hospital.

So let me start again. In France, at the start of my great adventure in July 2013, I was involved in a bicycle crash which resulted in a severe bang to the head. This means that I still cannot remember a large chunk of 2013. Even now I struggle to remember even the most mundane things about that blackout period. Occasionally something will shine in the darkness but it is mostly a featureless void.

So I apologise for the disjointed nature of this story. It is just a reflection of the way I remember things as in the early days after my crash, I lived a mismatch of experience and memory, and it felt almost like living out those fast-paced, sometimes confusing but always exciting comic books. If things seem a bit tangled up, I hope that you will take this sometimes rambling, occasionally disjointed and often brutally honest approach as an opportunity to see things from a different perspective and your chance to glimpse what it is like to have one's head all muddled up.

The next logical issue that might spring to mind about this story is how with such a deficiency in my memory I could put together something worth reading. If it was a true reflection of my slightly scrabbled head, the start of this story would be filled with many blank pages. Instead, to write the beginning of my story, I embarked on a detective exercise, putting the puzzle back together through the various appointments, tickets and adventures not had.

Apparently, it was all supposed to kick off in July 2013 with my triathlon training camp in the French Alps, culminating with the London triathlon, a pay-out for a year of hard work preparing my body to deal with the physical strain and my mind to overcome mental challenges. Then my planned great adventure was to begin. I had carefully managed my finances so that monetary concerns would not stop me doing anything (within reason) I wanted to do during my half-year off. Finally, money *and* time! This was to be my reward for my hard work, spending five years at university and five years with my nose flat to the grindstone at work. My first real break, as I had followed the path that every Chinese parent aspires for their children to follow – becoming a doctor or lawyer.

Although I had decided to follow this road with relentless drive, I soon found that there was a little problem with this approach. Everyone else was on it too. Apparently being a lawyer was a fairly popular pastime. It made the route very crowded, at times requiring a bit of force to move ahead. As I struggled to progress, after a couple of years I realised that I was getting a bit tired. This was compounded by an upcoming quarter-life crisis which made me think that I needed to do something noteworthy with my life. With this in mind, I planned some time off to visit exotic locations around the world. I thought that my extended vacation would not only help me build perspective but might provide experience and material for a literary endeavour. That could be my contribution to society, writing the story of a sarcastic, sometimes witty, but always deadpan lawyer.

As I completed my detailed plan for my time off, I realised that I had a bit of a blank spot in my diary right at the start. While searching for ideas of ways to pass the time, a worthy pursuit seemingly dropped into my lap as a friend passed along word of a training camp in France. In my slightly masochistic frame of mind, I eagerly signed up for this "holiday." I was seduced by the literature that marketed it as an idyllic place to train as the home of the famous cycling race, the *Tour de France*. Indeed, the training camp was to take place near one of the stages and at exactly the same time. This would provide plenty of opportunities to be spectators (or hecklers) of this Everest-like event in the cycling community. I would challenge myself through my own training and, in short interludes from such, cheer on others.

Little did I know that this casual and impulsive decision would come to redefine my life. At the start of my time off, I hopped over the English Channel to France to enjoy my two-wheel pursuits. Abuzz with energy, I simply couldn't wait to start my new adventure. Yet right at the very start of my time off, while pedalling peacefully along the picturesque French countryside, I fell on my face, spoiling my good looks. The rest of this autobiography is the exciting story of my new life.

The most exciting day of my life

As I lay there on the road with various fluids oozing out of me and my face a bloody, mangled mess, I must have presented a rather dramatic picture. Although I was in a coma due to the severity of the injury, amid the flurry of activity around me following the crash, inside my brain even more exciting things were happening. In such a sensational setting, with my various pieces of protective equipment now scattered in a more haphazard fashion than intended all over the road, began the most exciting day of my life. As a result of this electrifying event, I spent the next eight days in a coma.

From what I have been able to piece together, I understand that once the paramedics arrived at the scene they did some initial treatment and triage and determined that I would have to be evacuated to the nearby St Claude hospital as soon as possible. On arrival at St Claude hospital, I was hurried off to have a scan of my head and then, following discussion of the results, I was marked for urgent transfer to a tertiary specialist hospital as things were worse than initially suspected. I was then airlifted by helicopter accordingly to the regional Jean Minjoz teaching hospital.

Once I had been disembarked from the helicopter at Jean Minjoz, the doctors' main concern was treatment of the most critical problem, the fact that my brain was getting bigger and bigger. The initial shock of my facial contact with the road had caused a dangerous subsequent problem, my brain began to swell. Although swelling might not be a particularly dangerous issue when you bang your leg, with the brain things are a little bit more complicated as the skull is rather hard and inflexible. If the container cannot flex, the material inside will try to escape through the only viable opening in the skull, the spinal column. The concern was that the brain stem, controlling vital functions such as cardiovascular functions, might be pushed out of the head in such a situation. This process, called "coning," would lead to immediate death.

To keep careful watch on such a potential issue, surgeons then shaved my skull and inserted a transducer to measure intracranial pressure. This would give warning if things went from critical to dire. Even though my skull had not cracked in my fall, my "hard head" might have ironically been the end of me.

With this monitor now planted in my skull to provide early warning, the next step was to limit the expansion of my brain. To achieve this, strong drugs were administered to reduce the swelling of my brain. Yet such a procedure did not come without a cost. The drugs were so strong that they stopped me from breathing – things were moving from exciting to thrilling. Here modern medicine came to the rescue by providing a machine to breathe for me. Yet the dramatic story does not stop there. Another gripping side effect of such medication was that it caused my body's reflexes to shut down. This meant that I was slowly drowning myself. Under normal circumstances, the lungs will secrete liquid to self-clean and assist with functioning. With my coughing reflex rendered non-operational by the drugs, this normal and usually helpful bodily reflex became more problematic as my lungs began to fill with fluid. To prevent me from drowning, a more low-tech procedure than the complicated ventilator was employed – putting tubes down my throat and bailing out the lungs.

Thankfully all these activities took place while I was unconscious. Even imagining the trauma and pain makes me wince. I cannot envisage what the heart-stopping pain might have done to me. In this case, I think it is better not knowing.

Once I was a little more stable, at the end of my eight-day stint in the land of nowhere, I was slowly brought out of the grey fog. This was done very slowly as there was a significant risk that things could become even more complicated if not handled with appropriate delicacy. An abrupt reintroduction to the world had the very real danger of causing significant and additional complications; the shock might be too much. As an entirely expected consequence of this procedure, when the doctors tried to bring me out of my coma, I began to twitch uncontrollably. This was more than a slight issue as the spasms quickly spiked my body temperature to dangerous levels, so much so that I had to be subject to emergency cooling to stop me basting in my own heat. Icy water was circulated in tubes around my legs to get things under control. In an effort to further manage the problem, I was then quickly induced back into a coma. Once things were a bit calmer, another attempt to rouse me out of my coma was made. Unfortunately, this attempt was also unsuccessful. Several further attempts were made but the spasms just wouldn't stop. Instead, the doctors thought that it would be best to leave me alone as my body just needed a bit more time.

Once they managed to control the shaking, the doctors tried to wake me again. Now that I was a bit more subdued, through slow, staged movements, I was slowly brought back to the world of the living. As my essential bodily reflexes returned, the nasogastric (food) and endotracheal (air) tubes, central vein catheter (medication) and urinary catheter (pee) were slowly removed. Although this tubing saved my life, there was a risk that with so many foreign objects in my body, I might catch a secondary infection. I duly did so.

This was again an expected possible side effect so the doctors knew exactly what to do. The treatment would unfortunately be slightly unpleasant. A needle would be inserted into my spine while I was awake to extract the cerebrospinal fluid needed to diagnose the source of the infection. The pain of the needle punching into my spine was beyond excruciating. Through this sample and various other specimens, the source of the infection was determined. The applicable antibiotic was then duly administered through a venous catheter.

Now that I could move around without dragging half of the hospital with me and was nominally responsive, the story did not become any less exhilarating. Waking out of a lengthy coma was not like flicking a switch; the lights did not all suddenly come back on. Life was not as simple as the movies would have you believe. Coming out of a coma was a lengthy and fraught process. Some lights were broken and needed replacing. In other cases the transmitter and receiver were not talking to each other. With such problems, it was as if my wiring was ripped out. I wasn't able to function like a basic human being; I couldn't even remember who I was.

This memory problem was so profound that everyday life seemed almost comical at times. Even though I slowly regained a bare modicum of speech, there was a small cognitive issue. I was forgetting what I had just said a minute before, which made conversations exhilarating – for others, not me. I had no awareness of the things lost. I would not remember what I had just said and by the time I got around to thinking of the answer, I would have forgotten the question. Aside from this inability to hold up my end of a conversation, even more disturbing was that every time I drifted out of consciousness, whatever memories had managed to seep into my memory were lost as my life was reset. Now that I am able to look back, peering at my almost catatonic self, I know that in such a state every day was a repeating nightmare, a compounding state of confusion. From records of my early days and making presumptions based on my own nature, I am able to make a fairly accurate guess of what my then life was like. I would wake up in a room tied down, to prevent me removing all the wires and tubes stuck in me. In such a situation, I would struggle futilely and silently as I thought that I was being held hostage somewhere and needed to escape as quietly as possible to avoid alerting my captors. After much straining and effort, when I finally managed to undo any of my straps by wriggling and squirming, I would then find that I was not unobserved. The friendly nurse who was watching me would just do them back up. I would have screamed if I was able.

Even with such stunted memory, at the end of each day, just a little bit would have seeped into my mind, deep enough to stay for a while. Yet this was to be of little help as the biggest problem was that every time the lights went out, I started again from a blank page. Each time I awoke, I was forced to try and make sense of this almost unbelievable series of events. Yet when I finally managed to grasp what had happened to me through patient explanations, when I went to sleep I forgot it all. Each new day I would have to restart the process again. The most tragic thing was that I didn't even have an inkling that this had all happened before.

This memory issue would not be solved while I was in France, and the doctors decided that what was most important was to deal with basic physical function first. Once this was dealt with to their satisfaction, they deemed that it would be best for me to be transferred to a neurorehabilitation specialist hospital in London. The idea here was to wait until I was cleared for transfer so I would not suffer some urgent and potentially cataclysmic episode while in the air, a scenario in which help might be a bit difficult to deliver. I am told that this transit was quite exciting as I was loaded onto a specialised air ambulance designed to keep a low altitude. This was to avoid making my big head bigger as the pressure difference would play havoc with my damaged brain. Here I was reminded of empty water bottles I would take on a plane. At the end of the trip they would be thoroughly misshapen. I wouldn't want something like that happening to my head. Several hours later, I arrived in London without any mishap occurring.

Following arrival in London, the knives soon came out again. I underwent surgery to rebuild the right side of my face through the insertion of a titanium frame and the breaking and resetting of my nose line. However, there is nothing to see now as all the surgical additions are hidden under my skin, so you will need an X-ray to see my terminator-like visage. A friend remarked to me several years later, "Why didn't you get them to improve your face!" I explained that I had demurred as I preferred to be all natural. I wished to avoid any suggestion that I was not being open. I wanted people to be able to read the truth from my face and avoid any suggestion that I was hiding things.

The message from the various procedures I had endured seemed to be that medicine can do amazing things, but sometimes things just have to be left to prayer. Immediate critical physical injuries were dealt with in relatively straightforward ways, but other more complicated problems were not subject to such a quick fix. These problems ranged from the relatively minor, such as the loss of fifteen kilogrammes of weight and significant weakness on my left side, to the more material, such as the inability to walk, talk and remember. It was the latter that was to cause me the most trouble, even after I was out of the acute phase. Given the seriousness of this issue,

I think I would be remiss if I did not spend more time delving deeper into my memory issues. Although now out of my critical phase, with most of my fundamental memories somewhat intact, beyond this it was the great unknown. Some people rationalise memory loss as a defence mechanism of the brain, blocking out traumatic memories.

However, through personal experience, I can confirm that it is not so simple. When I woke from a coma, it took me several days fraught with worry before I could even recognise my parents. It was not as the media would have you believe, or as dramatic as the mental blocks experienced by adults due to some childhood trauma. Instead, it was actually far more ordinary and therefore even more heart-breaking in its effects. An insult to the brain (a bang on the head) causes retrograde (before the injury) and anterograde (after the injury) amnesia. For me it meant that I could not remember things from before my crash. Neither could I store memories of things that happened in the months after. My memory was like a revolving door. Nothing could stay inside. Everything went in one side, out the other.

As a subset of anterograde amnesia, I also suffered from post-traumatic amnesia, which is when the brain is unable to store events as they happen in memory. As a result, I would constantly restart conversations, repeating the same thing, having no idea that I had said it previously. I am able to relay the start of my story despite my memory problems as copious medical notes provided somewhere to start and a basis to seek further answers. The other way that I was able to relay the early days of recovery was to note "interesting" events in a small notebook. At first encouraged to use this medium by my medical team to help rebuild my concept of time, I later found it to be a godsend when writing out my story.

Sadly, memory issues are a somewhat misunderstood injury, despite strident efforts being made by individuals to raise awareness. It's not like in the movies where memory loss seems to be so clear-cut and relatively easy to live with. In reality, the far more damaging element is when the injury affects the future. Forgetting the past is very sad and crippling, but not being able to remember prospective events quickly brings you to a standstill as it leads to difficulties moving forward. From my perspective, with such memory problems, it seemed that life simply did not progress.

One particularly sad case of such issues is that of Clive Wearing, whose memory never recovered from his brain injury. His memory was limited to two minutes as described in his biography written by his wife Deborah Wearing, *Forever Today: A Memoir of Love and Amnesia* (2005). A particularly striking example of his memory limitations was contained in his notebook. In it were many entries with time references repeatedly noting that he was awake for the first time. His diary then showed proof of the disorder of his mind as he had crossed out his own writing again and again with entries that he was "awake now," "finally awake" and "truly awake!!!" Sadly, he had been stuck in this loop for many years and had no awareness of the recent past.

With such an acute problem affecting my everyday interactions, it proved a bit difficult to locate a suitable medical facility to treat me as, although the surgery could be carried out almost anywhere, the subsequent months of neurological care would necessitate careful thought. As a result of the type of damage wrought on me by my accident, in my early days out of a coma I could not remember what I had just done and had to have the past explained to me time and time again; my progress was glacial. I felt that I was constantly playing a game of catch-up, with the additional problem that the finish line seemed to move every time I blinked my eyes as I was summarily deposited back to the start.

This was not even taking into account the dangers that I posed to myself. As I was constantly in a state of confusion, there was a very real possibility of me walking out into the wider world and becoming lost in the general population. Therefore, special training and facilities are required to deal with patients suffering from memory problems. If that was not enough to think about, my condition was only exacerbated by the host of other commonly found ancillary issues. Such treatment centres are few and far between, but I was fortunate in that there was one in my home city of London – the Wellington hospital.

Here I ask for your forgiveness if my description of the immediate aftermath of my crash is relatively brief and circumspect. The circumstances surrounding my incident have been largely pieced together from various medical reports, my own notes and what other people have told me. Although some memory has returned, most of the months surrounding my crash are sadly missing. As I am not able to provide more detail, it might be useful if I instead take another step back to give a bit of background of my history. After all, it wouldn't do for you to not have the right perspective.

My boring history

As I was soon to discover, context and perspective would be key to recovery. My hope is that by sharing a bit more detail about my past, you will be able to understand my story a bit more fully.

In the beginning, I started my life in Sydney, Australia, the land of many dangerous critters such as koalas and kangaroos. Other less friendly creatures, like the redback spider, were not really for joking about though. As I was just finishing primary school, my family moved to Hong Kong following my father's medical profession. This was a far cry from the rolling suburbia of Sydney, with forests of skyscrapers instead of trees. In such an environment I was enrolled in high school. The atmosphere there was slightly competitive at times. Classmates would on occasion not be above competing with fervent vigour to get a single percentage point above their friends. By the time of my graduation from high school, I found that in such a combative environment I had managed to mould myself into a rather serious and solemn fellow, preferring books over physical activity.

Throughout my high-school career, team sports were abhorrent to me. Instead, I was encouraged to derive recreation from playing piano, which would also have the benefit of making me a well-rounded individual, broadening my horizons and increasing my attractiveness on my *curriculum vitae*. Being the obedient son that I was, I poured my efforts accordingly into music, quickly achieving recognition for my musical accomplishments at a very young age. This focus on musical talents also gave me a good excuse when people tried to convince me to come play ball. I would just say I needed to practice piano instead. However, this legitimate excuse masked another reason for my refusal: I disliked team sports because I was less than stellar at them. Because of my fiercely competitive nature, I simply did not like not being the best. Instead, I decided that sports would be put on the back benches for now and would be something I could concentrate on later.

The time for change came when I flew over to the United Kingdom to begin my tertiary education as transporting my piano overseas posed particular problems. A further reason to enthusiastically engage with team sports was that during my first period away from home I was presented with a chance to mould myself as I wished. No one would know who I was and I was unburdened by history; I could make myself into the sports fanatic that I had missed out on being. No one would know I was a less than willing participant in team sports in my earlier life, so I seized this opportunity with alacrity. With this chance to start from a blank slate, I then threw myself into sports.

A further reason why I had not participated in team sports as a juvenile was its element of danger. I never knew what injuries I might sustain when involved in such high-energy activity with others. Now that I did not have to pay meticulous attention to the care of my fingers to safeguard my musical skills, I thought that I was now free from constraints. Making up for lost time, I then founded my school's Ultimate Frisbee team, eventually building them up into regional champions. Not one to sit idly on my laurels, I also captained the university Karate team, winning awards and medals for my fighting spirit.

As I completed my tertiary education faster than I had wished, I then found it was time to start work. Thankfully the legal career path was fairly clearly laid out and I managed to secure a spot at one of the goliaths of the legal world in fairly short order. I felt that things were going exceedingly well at this point. I then spent a further year in practical training, learning how to be a polished, sophisticated and almost incomprehensible lawyer. With these prerequisites achieved, I then started work in the place of my dreams. I soon found that in such a high-stress job with demanding hours, the most useful thing I had learnt at university was determination, an unyielding spirit to never give up.

Following the start of my gainful employment, my recreational interests also changed. I loved the sporting activities I had pursued in university but they required extensive time commitments. So once work began in earnest, I thought I would need to engage in less intensive pursuits. I therefore changed to a less time-intensive and slightly less painful line of recreation: triathlons.

I found it much easier to compartmentalise my life this way as there were set limits to such a solo pursuit. As an individual sport there would be no friends to implore me to stay around for just one more lap, or just one more goal. Nonetheless, as with my other sport activities, I took it a bit too seriously; I would spend over ten hours a week concentrating on my cycling alone. Alongside this, I also worked on swimming and running, the two other components of triathlons. I found that this sport seemed particularly well-suited to professionals, as it was full of shiny expensive toys and competitive amateurs. Following the initial goading of my friends, before I knew it I had completed four triathlons. Amidst the pain, I later found that I actually rather liked it. These many factors led to me throwing myself into the sport wholeheartedly; not one for half measures, this obsession would easily eat up half my weekend. So much for managing my time.

In my entirely foreseeable and relentless pursuit of even faster times, I decided to venture to the French Alps to improve my cycling prowess. In my increasingly competitive frame of mind, I just had to outdo myself. A solo hobby was ideal as no longer would I be subject to the availability of others if I wished to test my mettle. I would only have to compete against myself, someone I could never beat, someone who would always be there to goad me on. Now that was perfect.

There were, however, some problems with competing against myself; it made things even more difficult as I couldn't lie to myself if I didn't perform. This meant that I would have little sympathy for myself when I did not reach my goals. If I did not surpass my own records, I proceeded on a course of metaphoric self-flagellation. I would know that I hadn't trained hard enough, lacked will or simply couldn't be bothered, and I couldn't accept excuses from myself. In hindsight, this slightly unhealthy obsession was how I ended up leaking various bodily fluids over a lonely mountain road. So began the most exciting day of my life.

The Wellington hospital

Although my emergency treatment was handled with great skill, aplomb and professionalism by the staff at St Claude and Jean Minjoz hospitals, my further rehabilitation would need to be dealt with at a specialist centre due to the complications of my severe brain injury. It almost seemed as though my multitude of problems built up into a wailing crescendo, a perfect storm, which could only be calmed with great difficulty. Following my repatriation to the United Kingdom by air ambulance, an exciting episode if I were able to remember it, I was installed in the Wellington hospital to deal with this trauma. This hospital specialised in the treatment of cases of traumatic brain injury. It was particularly well equipped and staffed to deal with the specific difficulties that head injury patients might display.

After a suitable interlude after my arrival at the Wellington hospital, I was visited by my supervising physician, Dr Richard Greenwood. I was later to find out that Dr Greenwood was one of the foremost neurologists in the world. This was the reason why my family had chosen the Wellington hospital, everywhere we had asked his name kept on popping up. It almost seemed fated that we were to meet.

I was later told that when I first met him I was extremely confused. Suffering from amnesia, I had no idea where I was or who I was talking to. As this was a common effect of an insult to the brain, the staff at the Wellington hospital were used to enduring the tedium of reintroducing themselves to patients each day. As part of my daily routine, each day I would be asked if I knew where I was to check if my memory was coming back. Although I had no conscious recollection of the answer to this question, the repeated introductions must have slowly seeped into my mind, as one day my answer instead of "I don't know, why don't you tell me?" was "We are in the Greenwood Hotel." After Dr Greenwood left, the remaining staff questioned me about who had just come to visit. "The general manager of course," I replied.

The next day, one of the staff couldn't help but ask during my morning orientation with Dr Greenwood who I thought he was. Apparently I replied while he was in the room that he was the general manager! Although I cannot remember the incident, based on my later recollections, I can imagine his very British reaction, a wry half smile. On the many later occasions I was to meet him, I would always find him particularly striking. It wasn't that he had a particularly interesting appearance, but rather that he seemed to fit the stereotype of caring, brilliant doctors. He seemed to be perpetually harried, with a slightly frazzled countenance, as if he were a brilliant scholar a step out of time; no time to pay minute attention to his appearance because he could be saving lives instead.

It was a good thing that I had a positive impression of the doctors at the Wellington hospital, as it was to be my home for almost half a year. I have the dubious distinction of having stayed at all three branches, the Platinum Medical Centre (day surgery and outpatient appointments), the South Wing (acute care) and the North Wing (rehabilitation). The staff became very used to me, no doubt helped by the fact that I was one of the few English-speaking patients. This strange oddity was a bit puzzling to me at first.

The Wellington hospital is located in leafy St John's Wood, just above Regent's Park, an affluent borough of London. Surprisingly to me, the general population of the rehabilitation wing where I spent most of my time did not reflect its location. I had thought that in keeping with the area, its patients would be genteel English men and women. This was not the case; the hospital population did not even reflect the national ethnic make-up of the United Kingdom. I think out of the fifty or so rooms in the rehabilitation ward, I was the only patient of Chinese descent. That was of no particular surprise to me, but rather more unusually I would soon also find out that the number of British patients could be counted on one hand, which I thought was slightly puzzling. Where did all the patients come from instead?

Just as with the make-up of London's property owners, a large number of the patients originated from the Middle East with a scattering from other places of the world. This made for quite an eclectic mix of patients and staff and posed its own challenges. In this almost United Nations of a hospital, reflective of many countries in the world, there were entirely foreseeable language difficulties. As many of the patients' native tongues were not English, the staff needed to be multilingual or skilled at mime. Most of the non-English-speaking patients spoke Arabic. Although there were several translators on staff, they could not always be there when needed. Staff would accordingly learn at least a smattering of Arabic along with accompanying wild hand gestures, making for crude but effective communication. Although the subtleties were sometimes missed, a combination of vigorous gesturing and the use of simple words served to prevent patients from eating objects that were not to be consumed.

Although there were particularly energetic attempts made to get the message across through whatever methods were available, sometimes it just wasn't enough. This meant that on occasion when the patients had been a bit too enthusiastic with the therapy putty, the therapists would need to dig play dough out of a patient's mouth. Although I found this particular task to be quite disgusting, it was preferable over manual evacuation, a duty dreaded by trainee doctors. It is as bad as it sounds and if you haven't managed to figure out what it is, I will not enlighten you. There are some places where the sun don't shine ...

Moving on from the description of the patients to the physical surroundings, the Wellington hospital prided itself on providing the best possible environment for healing. This was despite any cultural differences between the patients and the staff, as the doctors at the Wellington hospital were all, by and large, middle-aged British born and bred. The same could not be said of the therapists. The average age of the therapists in the hospital was relatively young, with most in their early- to mid-twenties. I assumed based on the accents (confirmed after some judicious prodding) that most were actually foreign nationals who had come over to gain a couple of years' neurorehabilitation experience in the United Kingdom. Fresh off the boat, the youthful optimism and cheeriness of the therapists in an area of so much sadness and pain was exactly what was needed. They would provide some much-needed sunshine to a rather dreary locale as one of the chief goals of the hospital was to provide the most conducive environment for healing. Connected with this was the emphasis on creating an understanding and supportive environment with staff that would emphatically avoid making any judgements on patients based on their present capacity as premonition of their degree of recovery.

Although the above description may lead you to think that the hospital was some type of hotel, there were subtle physical reminders that this was not a place I had willingly picked to spend my time off. There were no locks on any of the doors so that the staff could gain access quickly in an emergency. Panic buttons and cords were liberally sprinkled around, for those times when a patient might need assistance, and were also colour-coded depending on urgency. It did seem to me that the colour scheme was a bit nonsensical. I wondered, if you were about to have a seizure, would you have enough presence of mind to wonder which cord to pull? "Oh no, I am having a seizure. Do I pull the red or yellow wire?" The moment of indecision might lead to help arriving a little bit too late.

Entering on the ground floor, a visitor would not be remiss in thinking that this was some type of private club rather than a medical facility. There was a distinct absence of gurneys, brightly coloured medical personnel or wailing alarms. As a rehabilitation centre and not an emergency ward, time was not of the essence, but merely of pressing urgency. That is not to say that there was a lack of safeguards altogether. The reception was always manned, usually by three receptionists of whom at least two seemed to be of the stocky male variety. They were ostensibly there to provide assistance to visitors. Yet their real reason was to provide a final physical obstacle to any escape bids by patients.

Moving on to a description of the room, each was equipped with an en suite bathroom. A large TV was placed in a prominent position in the room, which also had an armchair for individual lounging (as much as you were able to kick back your heels and take your ease in hospital) or for guests. Interestingly, when I flicked on the TV to do a bit of channel surfing for the classical music channel to bring some peace to my room, there instead appeared to be a multitude of Arabic TV channels. No doubt this was in the belief that it would provide the majority of the hospital patients with a feeling of home. The low ambient noise of the hospital would also often be punctuated by the shouts and screams of the other patients or loud remarks from their visiting family and friends who were trying to cheer them up.

Attached to the ceiling of my room was another non-standard (unless you worked with livestock) addition. This was another clue to the real nature of my room. Called a hoist by the staff, it undoubtedly had some fantastically technical name created by the manufacturers to help it sell. Its true purpose was far more mundane as it was used to assist with the movement of patients. Depending on the individual, mechanical assistance would move from being helpful to essential.

This reminder was particularly apt as, at times during my hospital stay, I felt a bit like livestock as the various medical personnel would have conversations about me as if I was not there. Once during a conversation about me which took place literally over my head as I sat in a wheelchair, I waved my hands around and exclaimed, "I'm right down here you know!" Despite this outburst, I was still ignored. This failure to be heard was to later cause particular distress as further explored in "A second childhood."

The floor's material also gave another hint that this was not a holiday abode. It was not the plush carpet that you would expect in an upmarket hotel but consisted of plastic laminate flooring, easy to hose down if there was a "spillage" of any liquids, such as a little accident on the way to the bathroom. There were also an unusual number of card readers to prevent patients from making an unauthorised dash for freedom. On occasion, this "trap" would also snare unsuspecting staff that forgot their key cards and had to resort to frantic banging on the doors in the hope that they would not be mistaken for and ignored as an unruly patient. Instead, the hope was that a kind soul would rescue them from the delights of the stairwell.

Yet everything was not all fine and dandy or bright and happy, despite my attempts to put a brave face on at the hospital. It seemed almost counter-intuitive to me that the walls of the patients' rooms were actually somewhat thin, such that sound was allowed to travel relatively unimpeded. Either that or I was unusually sensitive to noise, perhaps because my sense of hearing became keener to compensate for my impeded sight. In the early days of my recovery, I only had one eye. With such a large part of the world missing, I felt a bit like I was entering my twilight years. Yet as I was reminded, one was better than none. On occasion, the nature of the patients' injuries would forcibly be brought to light; as in a desperate scramble to return to normality, patients sometimes tried to act as if they were on holiday. Maybe this explained the rather weird behaviour of some of the patients who were caught lighting up a joint when the staff weren't looking.

Other bizarre, or perhaps more understandable, behaviour displayed by patients included complaining about things. Not some things. Every. Single. Thing. As an example, one day I overheard another patient making a valiant attempt to discredit all aspects of hospital care and hopefully distract the hospital staff from continuing with the treatment he hated. Didn't they know not to keep on bringing in weird Indian food? Didn't they remember how many times he had said he hated Indian food? It reminded him of that horrible time at his post in the Far East. Horrible insects and stuff. Didn't they understand that the proper way to make a bed was to have the blanket folded down just so? What type of a hotel was this? Incompetent staff. Did the therapist have a husband? No? Need to have someone to keep you warm at night you know. What's a young woman like you doing without a man? So it went on. Continuously.

As for me, my way of dealing with things was not so vocal. It was to read. Thankfully I was saved from the selection of literary material as my brother had thoughtfully delivered my electronic reader to my bed one day. As I started to leaf my way through various titles, I later remarked to my brother that these books were exactly what I liked. How had he figured out I would love them? Was it some type of brotherly intuition? I didn't know he liked to read the type of books I did! As it turned out, there was an unexpected benefit to losing your memory. Who knew me best?

Well, myself. I had actually bought these books in the first place, sifting the titles to be left with the gold. It was almost as if I had had a personal shopper pick out exactly what I would like and deliver it to my bedside table. Once this realisation started to sink in, I tried to take some small comfort in the fact that even after my crash, my tastes had not changed too much. I should be confident that in my core, it was still me as I still loved the same things. I was still there inside, severely battered, bruised and missing chunks of flesh and memory, but still me.

My propensity to be a bookworm also had another small benefit. I would gradually build stamina in my arm by lifting up books and mental fortitude by imagining a different world in my mind. When things became too much, I would retreat into my own rosy world in my head. By indulging in this little bit of escapism I could pretend that everything was alright. I especially needed this when I was treated like a child, unable to make the right decision.

In such situations and with my mental state so compromised, my family stepped in to make my choices for me. They would schedule my appointments, decide on courses of action and even pick my food for every meal. Trying to see a positive side to things, I tried to view my stay in hospital as a character-building exercise. I should be grateful to have the opportunity to experience what it was like to grow up again. Now I would have the most excellent opportunity to repeat my formative years. I would have a chance to make my life different through this new start. Yet this great opportunity suffered from a not inconsequential issue. Due to my memory problems, it meant that I would be repeating my childhood again, yet without the benefit of hindsight. Instead, with my impaired memory, maybe the best analogy for my situation was not beginning as a baby again, but instead slowly failing from old age.

A second childhood

I have heard people say that when you grow old, it is as if you enter your second childhood. You need someone to wipe spittle from your face, feed you food and bring you to the potty. Having suffered an insult to the brain, I forgot how to do the most basic things. So in order to live, I needed to depend on others as if I were a baby again. Looking back now, I feel that it was an assault on my very dignity as I had to suffer the humiliation of having someone spoon me food like some drooling infant. What goes in goes out, so I also had to suffer the indignity of having someone wipe my bottom. Although I guess the silver lining is that I was unable to remember the ignominy of having to be treated this way, as my brain was still not wired correctly. Instead, the knowledge of what I had been through sunk in when I saw others treated this way. That was once me.

With a new baby, parents rejoice with their first word, their constant wide-eyed wonder at the world and their initial attempts to grasp at straws. For a child in a man's body like me, it was instead dispiriting for my parents to see me go through the learning experience for a second time. There was no joyful speculation that a rapid grasp of language pointed at a possible poet. There was no elated supposition that an enjoyment of water hinted at the next swimming champion. There was no wonder when I completed these milestones for a second time. Instead of excitement when I completed a task, there was a slight abatement of fear followed by apprehension of what could go wrong next. There was no reason for applause when I said my first word, only sadness that I found it so hard.

Yet when things went well in my recovery, I grew annoyed that things were not progressing fast enough. In such a state, I felt that I was constantly straining at the leash, like a child strapped into their buggy straining to reach for a shiny bauble. I wasn't allowed to touch things that were frustratingly put just out of reach for my own good. In my infantile state, I lacked understanding of why I was being held back. Yet time and time again when I reached too far and failed, the numerous episodes of defeat would be a brutal reminder that I really was still a child and a reminder that the slow progress was for a very good reason.

Later on when things were not physically beyond me, a well-meaning adult would stop me. I could see in their eyes that they thought they were protecting me from myself. As the frequency of these actions progressed, I found myself cringing and flinching away from such possible reactions, as they seemed to be reaffirmations that I couldn't be trusted to perform yet another basic task. It was a rebuke akin to parents telling a young child that the bike isn't for him, not just now but maybe forever.

Attempting to find my way out of this infantile state, I tried to assert myself by saying that I was ready, but would be discounted as not having the mental capacity to make an informed decision for myself. People around me thought that I couldn't know what was best for me in my reduced set of circumstances; the child should be ignored for his own good. Such reactions caused me no end of despair as it seemed that so many things were beyond me, never to be recaptured or experienced again. In the moments of my greatest despondency, I felt that the world just wasn't fair – it was purgatory to make someone relive the worst parts of their childhood without the balancing counterpoint of gaiety or laughter.

In such moments of sadness, it did cross my mind to hold a tantrum and hope that that would make everything better. After all, if I was going to be treated like a child, I reasoned that I should benefit from some leeway. Fortunately for others, before I embarked on this rash course of action, my growing awareness showed me that this would not be constructive. Instead, I displayed another juvenile trait, retreating into myself and sulking. After an extensive period of brooding, lasting weeks, I came to the realisation that I would need to control my flashes of rage and sadness. Instead, I would need to just concentrate on the here and now and stop worrying about my future. Acting like a brat really wasn't the way.

Even once I had grown mentally a bit, I still had many other hurdles to overcome. If a man is the sum of his memories, what was someone whose past was suddenly shredded? Something less? Even once I was able to nominally function, there was still the very difficult question of seeing how far I had fallen and how far my recovery might progress. To assess this, my every action was watched and questioned for clues as to my mental capacity. When my results came back, even if they were favourable, the next question was whether it was real progress or whether I had merely fluked. In particular, keen attention was paid to what I said as, to put it bluntly, they were trying to see if I made sense.

Having people listen to me was actually just what I wanted but for other reasons. Treated as an ignored child in those early days, I fervently wished that people would just pay attention to me. Even when it appeared like they were listening, it seemed that nothing was sticking. Instead, it felt like they were just going through the motions, but when I opened my mouth all they could hear was the wind. When they actually did pay attention though, I found that if they were losing they would have the ultimate trump card to play. They would say that I didn't know better. My decisions would be overridden as my fundamental basis for making decisions was suspect.

These actions made me feel marginalised as I could not be trusted to make my own way through life. That was actually not so far from the truth. When I was suffering in the hospital and things were not going as well as hoped, my family then stepped in to provide support as external help was needed. However, the well-meaning intentions of family ended up causing a great deal of conflict. I failed in many fundamental everyday tasks so they wanted to avoid troubling me with any decisions. They would make the choices for me, even if I wanted to decide myself. In such situations I felt as if I were watching my own life without the chance to influence it.

This family dimension caused significant upset. Although I could more easily see physical challenges such as walking/eating/breathing as an issue that would need to be dealt with as a natural consequence of an insult to the brain; dealing with family dynamics was completely unforeseen. I wished that someone had passed a word of warning here for family about the impact of brain injury on a loved one. I wished that they had been informed that they must carefully walk the tightrope of providing just the right amount of support, not infringing independence on one hand and not being seen as not caring on the other. Reversion back to an adult-minor relationship caused a great deal of anger, angst and sadness for all involved. I would rant at the over-protectiveness of my family as I thought I was a grown man, able to make my own mistakes. However, my family was protective because they felt that I didn't know what I was doing. With the benefit of hindsight, I now feel very sorry for my occasionally explosive reactions to family as for them it was like the blind feeling their way around for a dropped pin in a haystack, with the added complication that the focus of their attention would by turns become distraught and furious with their actions.

What was worse was that my family's well-meaning intentions sometimes made me feel as though my world was crumbling into dust. I thought that I should have been in the prime of my life. When I was in my late twenties with a stable job and in excellent physical shape, nothing should have been able to hold me back. To be thrust back into a parent–child relationship was traumatising for all involved. Yet, I have much to be thankful for from my family. Not only did they stand by me without any reservation and endure my ire, they worked tirelessly behind the scenes to make sure I received the best possible care when I could not fend for myself.

This was made even more apparent during my stay in hospital. Although the Wellington hospital is one of the best neurological rehabilitation centres in the world, with renowned medical staff, it still mattered very much who actually treated you as the actual rehabilitation was carried out by the therapists. Some of them were excellent, yet others seemed less so. In situations when things could be better, my family then returned to a role of looking after a small child. In my childhood state, even if I had the capacity to make complaints about my treatment myself, they would either be dismissed as not relevant, deranged ravings or meaningless complaints from someone who was not in an adult frame of mind. I was extremely fortunate that my family fought tooth and nail for me, composed as they were of an ideal make-up of professions, a doctor, a lawyer and a mother. Although outwardly I looked like an adult able to fend for himself, I very much needed family to hold my hand.

Even though it was best for me that they were there, I thought that it must have been far from pleasant for them. For my family, this situation had to be beyond their worst nightmares. Raising their son again from such a mental handicap with no guarantee of success was heart-rending, as was repeating the growing-up process which they thought they would never, should never, have to deal with again.

Over time, as I managed to attain a more adult frame of mind and was able to face the world more rationally, I was strongly advised that there was no shortcut to recovery. I would simply just have to retrace my life to attain normality. Hence, I had to endure the burden of growing up again. The problem with doing this a second time was that with some memory returning, and with the curse of history, when I failed I could see what I had lost. In such situations, despair would often come crashing down. In such circumstances, my emotions continued to switch so quickly between different negative feelings that they almost created a single mournful note.

What made things worse was that these feelings of bitterness and sorrow were compounded as my awareness of things missing grew. I came to realise that growing up for a second time would be even more difficult than the first as against the triumphs of milestones conquered there would be no rewarding elation. Trying desperately to find some positive element to my circumstances, I thought that I could now say that I know what the curse of omnipotence is like; I would have to grow up again without the heady joys of my first step.

The wheelchair and me

As one of the elements of building such formative experiences far ahead of my contemporaries, I had the bracing experience of learning what it was like to be bedridden. At the start, I couldn't even muster the ability to sit up in bed. Things just weren't working well. Several weeks later, once I was able to master the coordination to sit up and stay awake for more than ten minutes, the next stage awaited. I graduated to the wheelchair.

Once the initial burst of enthusiasm of being able to face the world upright passed, harsh reality started to sink in. Although I could now be conscious for more useful amounts of time, I was still disabled. From a wheelchair, the world was a cruel place. Now that I was able to move under my own power, it made me think about how in days gone by I would think that some of the saddest people I saw were those that were unable to walk. Now I got to experience this first-hand.

Yet even though I could now sit, walking was still far away. I was still too weak from my coma and the damage to my vestibular system, and I lacked the muscle because of bedridden-resultant atrophy to make the final transition to standing. It became abundantly clear why I needed the wheelchair. If I attempted tottering steps, the floor would come up to greet me without my permission. Even after I regained a bit of muscle, and was physically able to stand, the next problem was working on balance. I think you could refer to it technically as being "a little screwed up" as I would sway wildly from side to side. As my head had had enough trauma, I was keen to take it very cautiously to avoid banging it again.

This was a great contrast for me given my pre-crash life. It seemed so viciously unfair that just a couple of years ago in university I was in peak physical health. I had captained two of my university sport teams in winning numerous accolades and a significant haul of silverware. I felt that if I was determined enough and willing to put in the work, things would come naturally. At the time of my crash, I was in the best physical state of my life.

I was faster than I had ever been before. Yet now I was reduced to being an invalid. The disparity could not have been starker. Whereas I had once jockeyed for a gold medal on the sports field, now I struggled to move from my bed.

Such a lack of mobility profoundly damaged my self-esteem as it made clear to me how much I was dependent on others. Even though I was in a wheelchair, I still did not have freedom of movement. I was too weak to use my arms to wheel myself around, and so I still couldn't move freely. Instead, I was dependent on others' charity. I thought at times that it was such a merciless world that forced me to be so profoundly disabled. If I wanted to drink some water, I couldn't simply stand up and reach for my cup. It would be as out of reach as the top of a mountain. If I dropped something, it was as far away as the wreck of the Titanic on the deep ocean floor. If I wanted to go to the window to see what I had lost, it would be as far away as the North Pole.

Not being able to move under my own steam posed other difficulties. I could no longer do what I used to do when I was upset – storm off in a huff. Sanitary arrangements also proved problematic; it was difficult to use the bathroom when I could not make the transfer to the toilet throne. The hospital also contained other surprises. Slippery surfaces could turn my otherwise leisurely roll down the corridor into a velodrome experience, as I continued to pick up speed until I was rescued by a friendly hand or the less forgiving floor. The worst element of mobility woes was that at frequent intervals they would remind me of my disability.

Outside things were even more "interesting" as I could only venture into the wider world if I was gently pushed along by someone. I vaguely remember one occasion being wheeled around by my father. I thought that this was not something any parent should have to endure and I can only guess that it ripped into his soul. As he later told me, living with the continuous daily torment that something could go wrong was a process of protracted agony, a life with the constant apprehension that the pin would drop to reveal another problem. When I asked him if it was worse than burying his own child, he said that at least with death there would be finality and acceptance. Survival was in some cases a curse. This for me was one of the most striking moments of my hospital stay, an example of how much my invalidity was hurting others close to me.

As a laughably minor point, something else that bothered me was what other people thought of me. People might assume much about me if I couldn't stand. A man in his prime so obviously impaired, that poor dear, they might say, maybe he fell down the stairs? I didn't really notice the intense interest that some people showed in the mobility-impaired until I was the subject of their scrutiny. On my first visit to the outside community, being wheeled down the nearby high street by my physiotherapist, it was like entering a new world. Life experienced by a person in a wheelchair was quite different to that of an able-bodied man. While in my wheelchair, I noted that there were a variety of reactions to my invalidity. Some people would stand aside to let me pass. Others would be startled out of their daze when pondering what to have for lunch. The worst would be those that clearly noticed me but made no allowance for my reduced circumstance as they shoved in front or cut me off. After all, it's not hard to outpace someone in a wheelchair.

At times when I was in a temper, I would entertain thoughts of punishing those who made no allowance for me. It would feel so right to make them feel just a bit of what they were doing to me. Yet, the problem I realised was that the only threat I could carry out in my reduced state was to run over their feet with my wheelchair. Although this would give me a brief moment of glee, unfortunately, this was a little beyond me as I was already having so much difficulty moving down the straight and obstacle-free hospital corridors. It might prove slightly more difficult to master the necessary coordination required for this vengeful action. This was also completely ignoring any possible retribution that I would be ill-equipped to avoid. So, I had to content myself with dreaming of divine redress.

Trying to mitigate my temper, at times I entertained thoughts of how people would react if they were in my chair. Yet this came with its own host of problems as recasting things in this way showed that through my suffering I began to feel a sense of entitlement. When I felt that I wasn't given my "right" as a disabled man, the growing anger would quickly lead me into a spiral of self-pity. One particular example was when I was left alone by myself in the hospital corridor one day. I remember feeling waves of self-destructive thoughts. I was too weak to stand. I was incapable of rolling myself around. I was stuck in place as if glued to the floor and wholly dependent on others' charity. Sitting in my chair, alternating between bouts of self-pity and fitful rage, I came to the realisation that I could either wallow in helplessness or rise to the challenge. It was up to me how I wanted my life to play out.

Physical disability also caused other issues when I once became ill late at night in my room. There were emergency pull cords available for such situations. However, there was one small problem. I was too weak to leave my bed myself. So in this instance when I was feeling very unwell, I was unable to move the metre needed to reach the panic cord. Extreme distress then followed. Thoughts of being indefinitely stuck in this dependent position crossed my mind. In this instance, shouting, which later progressed to screaming, eventually had the desired effect. Someone came to my rescue, but not before I had managed to rub my throat raw.

Once I had managed to get over my grief at the loss of my former able-bodied self, my motivation slowly changed. It morphed from self-pity into a determination to escape the chair and the sympathy of others. I found it very distressing when I could see the condolences brimming in other people's eyes. My need to gain some measure of self-respect compelled me to push on despite the pain. At this stage, pride had replaced sadness as my primary impetus. When combined with anger at putting my family in so much pain, it was to become a more powerful incentive to walk, even more than my own personal pride.

With this change of mental attitude, my family saw that I would need a new teacher. The current one seemed afraid to push me too hard. With the goal of leaving the wheelchair in mind, my physiotherapist was switched to a fiery but sadistic New Zealander, henceforth referred to as the Kiwi. Together we made slow but steady progress towards unassisted horizontal movement. Previously, the physiotherapists seemed quite content to just let me bumble along without any real systemic change in my situation. Yet the Kiwi was something else. She was not content to let me coast along in an easy manner. She encouraged me onwards, but to do this she had to overcome my general apathy towards things. At times I just couldn't be bothered as everything seemed so hopeless. She had to find a way to motivate me.

I found that as the difficulty of our exercises increased, my urge to give up grew. To address this lack of motivation, she tried a variety of methods. Adhering to the doctrine of tough love, she would often cajole me initially with words when things seemed too hard. Her manner was so effective that as things progressed, she wouldn't even need to say a word to spur me on. Instead, only a raised eyebrow was needed to replace the unspoken words that she couldn't believe that a young man like me could have trouble standing.

Yet when this was not enough, she had many other weapons in her arsenal. When I bitterly complained about my invalidity, she rather bluntly said that if I didn't try, I would never know. She pointed out that I was acting like a spoilt kid. If I was going to be such a child, maybe I shouldn't be fit to leave the hospital. Did I really enjoy the hospital so much? Is the food so good here? Such harsh but true words compelled me to push on.

Supplementing this was a different approach, a direct emotional attack. She took a stab at my pride, reasoning correctly that moving to derision would touch on a nerve to push me onwards. The unspoken question that she raised through her judicial and sometimes sharp prodding was, "Did I really want to be like this forever?" She correctly reasoned that as I got better, what other people thought of me would become more important. As my recovery progressed well, what started to worry me was the thought that people who saw me in a wheelchair would assume that I simply lacked resolve and was too weak-willed to try and stand by myself. As a side benefit, once I managed to walk on my own, I thought she might stop harassing me. I might eventually be able to get a measure of peace.

The struggle and eventual triumph of unencumbered mobility did not come immediately, but was instead more measured as together we patiently grinded away at the various exercises in preparation for escaping the chair. Move the legs. Bend at the core. Hold the head just like this. Do it all together now. Before I knew it, the day when I bid farewell to the wheelchair was upon me. It would be one of the best days of my life. It was like I was back in university being awarded my medal for the university karate championships, except it was even sweeter. During my time in my wheelchair, I had often dreamed of escaping so I would no longer have to be dependent on other people's charity. No longer would I have to wait for others. No longer would I have to subject my family to daily torment.

In the way that most good things seem to happen to me, this day arrived without fanfare or heralds. There was no build-up or warning that something momentous was going to happen to me. It wasn't a big event like some attempt at the world record. The situation was far more mundane.

One day when I was sitting in my wheelchair, ruminations going through my head, I felt an urge to visit the bathroom. So I did what I usually did, which was to implore the nearest therapist for assistance. On this particular day I was in class with the physiotherapist. Braving the possibility of verbal derision, I asked her if she could take me to the toilet. I just needed to go that bad. In hindsight her answer was very much her attempt to goad me on, but seemed a bit blunt and lacking in compassion at the time. The answer from the Kiwi was, "Do it yourself."

So I did.

Standing on two feet

Once I had managed to regain my mobility and be a little less morose about life, the intensity of my therapy increased dramatically. I guess the idea was that if the therapists would not have to deal with the patient's angst and physical immobility, it opened up new vistas of treatment opportunities. Now that I was a bit more stable, I was ready for a change. As I was now able to participate in more cognitively demanding sessions without drifting off, my physiotherapy treatment was supplemented by occupational therapy – learning how to live in the real world; speech and language therapy – learning to communicate with the wider public; and neuropsychology – learning how the brain underscored every action.

Scheduling all of these sessions into my ten waking hours proved to be a logistical challenge. I would also be competing against all the other hospital patients for resources. Even once I was deemed a worthy investment for this amount of therapy, the problem was trying to fit it all in between multiple conflicting schedules. To deal with this, the hospital had an unusual approach. Every Friday all the therapists would meet together to thrash out each patient's schedule for the week. Finding the ideal balance between a frustratingly unattainable goal and too many elementary lessons was an exercise in finding poise on a carpet of marbles. Evidence of this horse trading was readily apparent on my weekly schedule as there were many crossed-out entries scribbled over with different coloured pens.

As I was unable to stay awake for prolonged periods of time, my schedule needed to be packed to make the most of my waking hours. The problem was that sometimes it felt so crammed that it was a bit too much; sometimes all I wanted was to be left alone. I felt that I needed time to think and mourn my lost life, but the intensity of my sessions often left me without the energy to feel sorry for myself. In hindsight, maybe this was the whole point. I wouldn't be given the time or energy to sink into recriminations of my past choices.

After I had learned to walk, my physiotherapy sessions changed. Although I had the same teacher as before, we now moved on to more advanced goals, such as learning how to move at a brisk pace. As these goals were slowly realised, the dark miasma around me began to recede. Now that I was not constantly in a state of depression, I found a little of my pre-crash personality reasserting itself. I tried to give a little back. To this end, I thought that maybe the hospital staff were entitled to a little entertainment of their own. They worked in an environment where misery was the status quo and laughter a scarce commodity. With this in mind, I enlisted the support of the sadistic Kiwi physiotherapist. Together we planned a little surprise. When she was to be on leave, I was to have a replacement physiotherapist. We settled on a challenge to see if I could reverse the roles usually played out in the hospital, to make the therapist the patient. Now we just needed an enthusiastic (and gullible) target.

So began the most entertaining day of my life in hospital. On the first day with the replacement, I said hello and exchanged the usual pleasantries with her. Having answered "I'm fine," it was then time to get down to business. Much as a frog would jump out of a pot of water if it was suddenly brought to a boil, I decided to start gently at first to avoid causing too much suspicion. As part of my usual sessions I would often be sent up and down the stairs to challenge my balance. When I feigned ignorance, she patiently demonstrated. As she was keen to point out, looking all around while descending was a very bad idea. You might go down a bit faster than you were intending. She declined to provide a demonstration of the likely outcome of this lack of awareness despite my protestations that it would help with remembering.

The next stage was to engage with the treadmill. When I convinced the replacement to show me how to run on a treadmill, I decided to demonstrate the special surprise I would customarily get from my usual sadistic physiotherapist – slamming the stop button, forcing an emergency deceleration. This was ostensibly to test my balance, but she later admitted it was mainly for her own amusement. The replacement did not share my hidden mirth when I aped what I had seen. Although, as I reminded one of my friends when she came to visit me later in hospital, you can't be mean to hospital patients. What would the rest of the world think of you? You might gain a reputation for bullying people who were in their most vulnerable state.

I managed to make it to day three before the replacement physiotherapist finally managed to put two and two together and simply refused to play along. Most of my other therapists were in on the joke and could be seen glancing around corners and smiling when they saw said replacement stalking the ward in a temper. When my original physiotherapist reappeared, she couldn't help but laugh that I had succeeded far beyond her wildest dreams. She also let me know that the tale was making the rounds of the hospital as well.

The other disciplines were not ignored but were much harder to quantify progress in. Although it was easy to see that I was making substantial gains in physiotherapy, thus allowing me to engage in a bit of humour, occupational therapy preparing me to survive in the real world suffered from a critical problem. Although the basics of living could easily be taught, measuring my occupational capacity was far more difficult. It was a challenge to pinpoint where I might next fall down.

In an attempt to address the former, living independently, the hospital staff would set me loose on the public at large by asking me to go here and do that and go there and fetch that, all the time under the watchful eye of one of the occupational therapists. The idea being that the real world without safety guide rails would be the ideal test. Yet this task was fraught with its own complications. I could misplace myself in the great wide world as a real risk for brain injury survivors is getting lost. Although hyper alert to such situations, on one occasion I still managed to lose the therapist for a prolonged period during one of my errands. I was in a shop that apparently only had one entrance at the front. I then left the shop unobserved by the not-so-prominent rear exit. When the therapist poked her head around to see what was taking me so long, I was nowhere to be seen. Panic then ensued. Luckily I was to reappear before the frantic searching escalated to yelling my name in public.

In addition to such daily tasks such as shopping and not getting lost in the city, occupational therapy would also deal with my return to work. While the therapists were racking their brains for something that would simulate my legal occupation, they decided that a short presentation to a small group of hospital staff would be appropriate. In an attempt to generate enthusiasm for the task, they asked me to pick a topic I was interested in. I decided that it would be instructive to make it on perspective, in this case, literally, the view from a camera. I thought it would be a suitable choice as it had many parallels to my own situation and my different perspective on life due to my eye injury.

I thought that such a topic would be suitable to my circumstances as brain injury exposed me to a radically different point of view. In this presentation, I planned to explain how shifting your perspective could make all the difference in the world to a photograph. An unidentifiable pillar in the distance could be easily identified as a bell tower from another angle; the seemingly nonchalant manner of the tightrope walker was even more amazing when a different point of view exposed the great drop beneath him; and the reason for a young man's lack of speed would be revealed when glancing down and noticing his strapped-up leg.

Yet an additional hurdle that I would have to overcome to do this presentation would be my stage fright. I have always been nervous about public speaking and was even more so in my first "public" appearance since my crash. While I started off my presentation well, I soon tripped up as an issue came to light – an inability to inhibit myself when I found the people staring at me to be a hilarious sight, so much so that I was unable to stop laughing for a full minute, even though it was obviously not very funny. To clarify here, they were not making funny faces but just listening with rapt attention to my presentation. I would commend my audience in this case for showing no adverse reaction to my loss of control. At my debriefing, this failing was quickly skimmed over. However, to me it seemed like a critical problem, perhaps hinting at my serious underlying deficits. There seemed to be much farther for me to go before I could be let out of the hospital.

The third limb of my rehabilitation was communication. Termed speech and language therapy, or SALT as they preferred to refer to it, it went beyond what I initially understood to be communication. SALT encompassed all communicative media, beyond the obvious verbal elements. It included subtle elements such as eye contact, hand gestures and an ability to maintain attention. SALT was crucial in my particular case as it would address one of my largest self-perceived failings, a loss of eloquent language. However, it was decided that at my then current stage of recovery, more acute issues needed to be addressed first.

Treatment of my ability to articulate myself in diverse ways would start slowly. First it would be important to ensure that I could chat about the weather. As I explain further in my chapter on "Understanding and feeling," I showed none of the usual facial expressions when I spoke. This caused some difficulty when talking to normal people, as they would either think I was bored with them, arrogant or simply did not care. This could prove problematic when interacting with the outside world. As it was explained to me, all of the almost involuntary movements, such as smiling when someone else talked or other little facial movements conveying attention, required conscious effort until you did it so much that it became almost natural. Although I was conditioned when growing up in the use of these social mannerisms, following my accident, making these efforts tired me significantly. However, as it was explained to me, these small expressions were invaluable to human communication. Out of curiosity I tried talking to the wall to see what it would be like. I soon gave up.

Through repeated practice and feedback, I slowly began to grow out of my zombie phase and came to appreciate the small elements of human interaction. In some cases, however, I thought that actually lacking any facial tells was an advantage as at this stage I would have made an excellent poker player and could provide a deadpan delivery of jokes. As I explained to one of the therapists when she questioned this, the entire premise of irony (as I pointed out, a very British type of humour so ideally suited to my environment) was to make off-colour remarks in a neutral tone that made it harder for other people to tell if you were joking or not. Likewise, keeping your silence could also be part of your comedy routine, seeing people grow more and more uncomfortable as they struggled to guess if you were telling a joke in the absence of any tells. My therapists did not find this funny.

The final part of my therapy was the most challenging – neuropsychology. This was education about why I was facing particular difficulties in life. It helped to put things in perspective as, for example, it wasn't that I was too dim to complete a task, but may have been because I just kept on forgetting steps. Ordinary life in itself was quite complicated and it only got worse when things didn't seem to stay where I left them. Neuropsychology helped me put in place strategies to mitigate my deficits. I was to carry around a small notebook and pen to help me remember things. As I got better and didn't strictly require pen and paper anymore, it became my little security blanket. An additional benefit was that it also helped me to declutter my mind. As it was explained to me, the brain is a very messy place. It might say, for example, remember to pick up the dog from the vet on the way to visit your parents. But also remember to pick up some milk from the stores. Oh, and it's also probably best to shine your shoes before going out. Being able to compartmentalise these tasks and write them down helped me to calm the storm in my mind.

Neuropsychology also dealt with the way that I viewed myself. Here the line between psychology and neuropsychology seemed to break down as treatment seemed to fall under both of these umbrellas. As an intrinsic part of this, neuropsychology also dealt with emotional issues. Dealing with my anger and sadness, my therapists tried to gently steer me towards a new sense of self. The sessions concentrated on helping me to come to terms with my new life and an understanding that although life would never be the same, the slide into depression should be best avoided.

One particular aspect that neuropsychology tried to address was my perspective. I was gently but persistently guided towards seeing that things were actually not that bad. I could at least walk around, talk (mostly) intelligently to people and live a fairly uninspired but mostly unfettered life. However, one of the neuropsychologists made an almost fatal error in saying words which seemed to undo much of the good work done so far: "It could be worse. You have so much to be thankful for. You can walk, talk and think." What followed was a violent backlash internally, as at this point I still couldn't accept my new self. What I did not need to hear was some exposition from others about how I had avoided further tragedy. I was knee-deep in self-pity and terror and did not need anyone to attempt to make soothing explanations. How dare they attempt to say I should make the best out of my situation? Who were they to pass judgement? Could they honestly say that things could be worse? Well, I guess I could be them.

At this stage it seemed almost as if I viewed the world in a rather flat, uncomplicated and too simple way. After this incident, my therapists realised that I needed to calm down a bit more before neuropsychology treatment could progress. Yet this wasn't something that they could actively help with. They could prepare me with all the tools I might need to progress, but it would be up to me to make use of them. I would have to take the plunge and plumb the underlying depths of my understanding and feeling and battle my own demons myself.

Understanding and feeling

Whereas it was relatively straightforward to treat and assess my physical progress, mental and emotional improvement was more difficult to measure and rectify. With the emotional aspect, the issue was that this had no easily foreseeable milestones to aim for. It was too abstract for that, and it was not as simple as appreciating that I couldn't stand and then understanding and treating the underlying physical issues that made an upright posture impossible. Instead, mental and emotional failure would be shown by my inability to complete activities unimpeded by physical infirmities.

One day in hospital when I managed to find a mirror, I took a long, hard look at myself. I thought that I actually looked pretty much the same as before. It was inside that things were quite different though; most of the damage was hidden out of sight in my head. My mental immaturity was not shown by a glance at my outside appearance, but rather by actions completed and not completed. Unlike a person with obvious physical infirmities, I did not walk around with a sign around my neck saying "recent victim of a crash, make way." The crux of the problem was when I failed at elementary tasks, I felt that the shining epitome of example I had built my premorbid self into was crumbling into dust.

My pre-crash self was particularly self-content. My satisfied self thought he had academically distinguished himself by completing a rigorous and difficult education to peer-reviewed recognition. He had also succeeded at some of the highest levels of sport, winning peer accolades. To top this all off, he then pulled it all together to professional acclaim by achieving a coveted position as a young, hotshot lawyer in one of the world's largest law firms. It seemed that nothing could stop him.

This made the ferocious crash even more excruciating. I had fallen from the top of the world to the hard earth below. It was as if I was not just knocked down a few pegs, but that the entire ladder had been shattered. As bleak as this picture seems, there was worse to come. Due to limited self-awareness, I didn't know that the game had changed.

At first I couldn't understand that I was different. When I tried to do easy sums in my head, I couldn't understand why I couldn't grasp the numbers. When I had difficulty finding the correct word for basic objects, I was stumped at my seeming ineptitude. It was not clear to me why I had such issues. I lacked understanding and recognition of the damage wrought on me. This lack of self-awareness proved to be a particular stumbling block to addressing my mental deficits.

At the mental stage of recovery I had reached by the end of my stay in the Wellington hospital, although I was not accepting of the deficits I had, I had quickly reached intellectual awareness of the same. As was later explained by staff at the Oliver Zangwill Centre, a specialist neurorehabilitation centre I was to visit, described further in "The Oliver Zangwill Centre," I knew quite well the textbook description of my deficits but lacked a "felt" sense of the impact, that is, how it affected me personally. At first this seemed like rubbish; of course I would be best able to judge the effect of problems on myself, as I obviously lived with myself unceasingly. However, I was also very aware that I could not provide an objective assessment of myself, much like I couldn't (unless I was rather fragrant) smell myself. I was just too invested in myself to provide a detached objective perspective.

I just could not, would not, accept that I was different. I could not "feel" the difference. I refused to accept I was a changed man after the crash. What made this a critical problem was that if I couldn't understand how my deficits affected my life, it would be almost impossible to try and mitigate issues that I refused to acknowledge existed in the first place. So in an effort to try and address this lack of awareness, my therapists painstakingly tried to make me recognise the real me in the mirror.

Through various therapy sessions and self-study, I learned that there are several stages to dealing with metacognition (the comprehension of brain injury). Beginning at the bottom of the awareness ladder, the lowest stage is "intellectual awareness," where I knew how injury to the brain would affect a person but was unable to appreciate it personally; I was able to see the problems in others but not myself. The next stage is "emergent awareness," which is explained as the ability to see problems as they might arise, a bit like a juvenile learning that chocolate is good to eat but that eating too much is a bad idea. The final level of awareness is termed "full anticipatory awareness," which was described as the ability to proactively make plans to deal with potential issues. In this example it might be as simple as mitigating temptation by setting a monetary limit so that the money would run out before things could escalate.

I found that my intellectual awareness was speedily achieved. I was soon able to demonstrate that I could quickly rattle off the medical terminology related to my injury and the usual consequences thereof, but failed to relate the effects directly to my personal circumstances. At this stage, I thought that I would make an excellent neuropsychology student. Although I was able to grasp the intellectual teaching with alacrity, it took a bit longer for me to progress from intellectual to emergent awareness.

In this next state I could partly see a way to return to a normal person, even if it was obscured by the clouds at times. In my emergent awareness state I was able to see some problems and plan around difficulties. Although, as time went by and I found trouble with some of the activities I had prepared for, I began to understand that there were hidden problems that I couldn't recognise. At this stage I was halfway there. The goal then came to avoid the hidden menace of the iceberg with its submerged eviscerating threat hidden out of view beneath the surface.

Over time, as I made peace with my emergent awareness, I then progressed to the final stage of metacognition, full anticipatory awareness. Growing out of a state of fastidious planning of every step I would take, I moved on to a more workable arrangement. I still carefully planned out my actions as far as I could but was not afraid to wing it at times. Thankfully my understanding of metacognition was to come relatively rapidly during my hospital stay. Acceptance on the other hand was a whole different ball game.

The second parallel process sitting alongside metacognition is acceptance, a more tricky issue to address as it is intrinsically emotional. In a similar way to metacognition, this process is also divided into stages. The first stage is no acceptance, a state of denial that anything is wrong. The next, partial acceptance, is the feeling that there is something off-kilter with the world, that things are not quite right. The final stage is full acceptance, understanding that there are some things that I couldn't do anymore. It was this final stage that was most difficult for me to accept. It was a very bitter pill to swallow. My journey along the acceptance pathway was particularly slow and painful.

At the start, I had no acceptance. I was adamant not to accept things were different. I was in a state of denial that the crash had changed me. When people asked me if anything was different after my crash, I would quickly reply that of course nothing was wrong. That is, except for some obvious physical issues, like the patch over my eye, the scars over my body and the metal plate in my head. Couldn't they see that there was nothing materially different with me? It was not like I was on life support or would have to be spooned food like a drooling infant. I would insist that I was pretty much the same person. Yet despite or perhaps sometimes because of people saying otherwise, I persisted in my self-delusion. I could not, would not, accept that I was different. I just couldn't see it and would not believe anyone who said otherwise. I needed hard proof.

It would take a demonstration by hospital staff to progress further along the acceptance journey. They decided that the most straightforward way for them to show me that I was different was through my speech. To that end, my therapists videotaped me reading back a passage and carrying out a contrived conversation with them. I was then shown videos of others who had speech problems following a brain injury and was asked what I thought was wrong with them. I was able to easily point out the speech impediments that they displayed with the benefit of the laborious explanations that my therapists had provided in previous sessions. After I had finished identifying the problems of others, I was presented with a video of the task I had just undertaken. We then played a game of "guess what's wrong with you." I was rather agitated as it became readily apparent that I displayed many of the attributes that I had readily identified in others. The major issue that I identified with myself was that talking to me was like having a conversation with the wall. I lacked any emotions, gestures or facial expressions and sounded like a computer, so monotone was my speech. I would have made an excellent voiceover for GPS systems, "turn right at the next junction and then continue one hundred metres until the second junction."

These exercises forced me to finally admit that I was different now; I had now progressed to the partial acceptance state. This was particularly valuable as now that I admitted that I was a little different, more effective treatment could be administered. To address this lack of modulation of tone, I was encouraged to imitate one of my Irish therapists who had a rather expressive voice. I was instructed to imagine that my everyday speech was an exercise in clearly enunciating my every word. One of my tasks was to treat this speech problem by greeting everyone I saw in hospital with a bellow of "HELLO!" I initially startled some of the staff but they soon became used to me using them as part of my therapy. Starting from such boisterous beginnings, I was assured that by a process of osmosis my ordinary speech would become a bit more captivating.

Yet even with such a dramatic demonstration of my deficits, the final hurdle of full acceptance still eluded my grasp. Although with the benefit of hindsight it was blindingly obvious that I was different, the little man in my head was unwilling to accept this reality. He just thought that he was slightly different from before, not significantly so but just a little. He vainly and childishly thought that if he closed his eyes and shut out the world, everything would be better when he opened his eyes again. Although my SALT treatment seemed rather trivial at the time, it had an important secondary objective – gently bringing me to realise that there might be the possibility that there were big differences in my post-crash self, thus working towards the end goal of full acceptance. Working on this theme, the SALTs continued my language treatment.

After settling the intonation issue, the next step was to engage in exercises to try and restore my use of non-verbal actions, that is, body language. I found that it was not the bigger emotions and gestures such as disgust and anger that were difficult for me to display, but rather the more subtle positive ones. The small but important little elements of appropriate eye contact, body position and affirmative movements were demonstrated as being key to being able to function in everyday life. They would be pivotal in convincing people to speak in anything more than social pleasantries with me. In contrast to the video sessions previously discussed, the lessons in this case were provided more directly. Through live demonstrations I was shown by the therapist what it was like to be very uncooperative, emotionless and non-communicative. When I questioned why I should even bother to pretend to be interested when I was not, the reply was what did I think their job was like? I conceded that this was a fair point.

Supplementing my work on learning body language was learning to empathise with people again. Although this sounds easy for most people, this was hard for me as I had been exposed to extremes of negative emotions. As a defensive mechanism I found that I had fenced off my ability to feel anything positive. I thought that I had more than enough issues to deal with myself and didn't need anyone else's troubles to add to that. The other connected issue was that I simply couldn't see how showing emotion could be anything more than a minor inconvenience. Although intellectually I understood that I would need to deal with emotions to inform my mundane everyday personality, I was simply unable to accept it.

I thought that there were much bigger problems to deal with. What about my eye? I still couldn't see half the world! The emotional rubbish of others could wait until much later, and I couldn't see how empathising with others would help me to heal. In my infantile state, learning to reopen my sensitivity to others was extremely difficult. I simply couldn't care less about how others felt; it was more demanding than learning to walk, more challenging than learning how to see and harder than learning how to laugh again.

For someone starting from absent emotions, I found pretending to empathise with others more arduous than climbing a mountain. Yet, empathising with others (or at least seeming to) would be critical to my mental and emotional development. As part of my rehabilitation, I was taught how to *show* emotion. Although I complained that I did not feel anything most of the time, I was instructed to just fake it even if I didn't feel it. I was told that it really didn't matter if I didn't feel anything. I would instead be learning as small children did, aping the expressions of their betters. Not unexpectedly given my recent experience, I found extremes of negative expression much easier to show, such as sadness and anger. More difficult was displaying positive emotions as, frankly, I could not muster the requisite enthusiasm.

My arrival at full acceptance could only be achieved when I could feel the full spectrum of emotions. It would not be good enough to just feel like I would cry as I would also need to learn rapturous joy. So in an attempt to try and address this unhealthy lack of positive emotions, my therapists played a game with me. I would be given a card with an emotion written on it. I would then have to act out said emotion. The therapists would have to guess what I was feeling. When I first participated in this, I adopted what they thought was a neutral expression when handed the card. The therapists then started guessing. Predictions ranged from happy to bored and excited. When they gave up and looked at the card, it read amusement. They complained that I did not seem amused at all. However, I explained that that was not true as I derived a great deal of hilarity from their futile probing. They did not find that funny.

As much as I complained that these exercises seemed childish, stupid and meaningless, they were gentle attempts to try and rebuild sensitivity to positive emotions. Nonsensical and fake as I found my exercises to be, I discovered that the way to relearn emotions was by pretence. By acting happy, amused, excited or interested, I could slowly grow to genuinely feel that way. As is explained by C.S. Lewis in *Mere Christianity* (1952), if you act in a hateful manner to particular people, you grow to hate them more and more. Thankfully the opposite is also true. Treat others as your good friends and they will slowly become exactly that.

As a further part of this particular line of treatment, I was asked to read a series of jokes to one of the therapists and make them laugh. I managed to achieve this, but not because of the meaning of the joke itself but rather my deadpan delivery. It was easy to be a comedian if you didn't manage to find anything funny. From here the progression of the task was to involve the wider hospital staff. I was then tasked with delivering a joke to the unsuspecting world. With my SALT hiding around the corner, I approached the matron and asked her if she could help me with a question. "What do you get from a pampered cow?" I asked her. When no useful answer was forthcoming, I told her "spoilt milk."

As part of this goal of progressing to full acceptance, I also had to develop my understanding of the abstract. This meant learning how the real world worked as a common effect of head injury was a concrete way of thinking. This medical term was shorthand for referring to the inflexibility and intractability of a person following a bang to the head. As a result of my crash, everything became literally literal for me. Wait a minute became just that. A promise to definitely get back to me about something became an ironclad guarantee. I would take things at face value and feel betrayed when people did not do as they said. Seeing my distress, one of my therapists gently reminded me that people did not actually mean what they said sometimes. It wasn't that everyone wasn't being truthful, but rather that I did not understand metaphors or similes. When people said that recovery would be like sailing solo across the Atlantic, they did not actually mean that.

To try and test my progression in understanding the abstract, I was periodically examined through the proverbs test. In this I was presented with many cards printed with various sayings. The task would be for to me to explain what these actually meant. As these lessons would be repeated as part of an ongoing process, I asked why we had to keep on doing them. Apparently the therapists needed to continue to test my ability to deal with the wider world. If I couldn't understand the abstract it might cause slight issues. If I took a favourite colloquialism such as "to be honest" at face value, did that mean that people had been lying to me before?

In an attempt to clarify the nature of the exercise, I queried when the therapists' worries would be assured away. They said that I should be able to interpret all the sayings before this particular line of treatment would be complete. I thought that this was ridiculous and voiced such thoughts. It would be impossible for someone to know so much unless they had devoted much effort to the study of such idioms. I voiced such concerns loudly. Did they know the meaning of all the sayings? People in glass houses shouldn't throw stones. They stopped soon after I said this.

Yet even after all this work, I was still not able to reach full acceptance. Like a child, I refused to accept the unwelcome reality. This view of life was appropriate to the mental stage that I was at. Although I had grown in leaps and bounds in mental age up to this point, as a mental juvenile, I still had not reached the point of understanding that kicking and screaming does not work. Instead, I needed to understand that logically my energy could be used far more productively to solve problems that I faced instead of resisting futilely for no apparent gain. Unfortunately, in this case, one particularly premorbid trait shone through to my detriment, my determination to do it my way. A less charitable way of referring to it would be stubbornness.

Thankfully through relentless application of lessons day in, day out, I slowly came closer to full acceptance. It just took a bit of time as the progression along the journey of acceptance could unfortunately not be subject to a quick fix. It would continue to underscore much of my treatment. Wearing away patiently at my view of the world and myself, my SALT sessions showed me how things were different, not necessarily any better or worse, but just different. A major breakthrough in this journey of acceptance was when I understood that it did not mean tolerating a life of reduced circumstance. It did not mean stomaching the label of "disabled." It was instead recognising reality and the emotional appreciation that things had changed. This did not mean that I shouldn't try and overcome my problems. It was not creating artificial barriers to recovery. Instead, it was just realising that life would be different.

The Bleakness

Unfortunately the return of my emotions was not without consequences. Now that I had been tutored to feel things again, I got to experience the full spectrum of emotions. Not only could I feel happiness, wonder and joy, but the contrasting emotions of disappointment, dismay and misery. These negative feelings pointed to a serious emotional dilemma; I could not understand why things had happened the way they did.

During spare moments in hospital, I found myself in a state of great conflict and confusion when I tried to make sense of what had happened to me. Thoughts would rush through my mind. Had I done something to deserve it? Was it something I had not done? Was it part of some little cosmic joke? When pondering this sad state of affairs, I found myself growing by turns sad, taciturn and then angry. I was later to learn that my internal debate closely mirrored the classic symptoms of dealing with grief. I would have the interesting experience of going through the stages of denial, anger, bargaining, depression and acceptance a little faster than I would have preferred.

Trying to rationalise why I felt so hopeless, I tried to seek the genesis of the pain. After much internal debate, I managed to pinpoint the crux of the problem; it seemed as though all my dreams were snuffed out in an instant by the crash. Against such a backdrop, on my worst days there seemed to be a lack of reason to keep living. In less mournful days, I would just be resigned. On the best days, I couldn't care less. Although on such better days I might lack gut-wrenching desperation, in such a state I still could not envisage a happy ending to my journey. As more and more issues came to light, at times it seemed like a never-ending nightmare. It seemed that I would be forced to try and make sense of increasingly more distressing situations after I had made peace with the latest tragedy.

I was told initially that I may never be able to see properly out of one eye, so I should make peace with half the light of the world. I was also softly prepared for the reality that I might never walk again, so I should practise my wheelchair skills. It was gently broken to me that I might end up living on indefinite support, so I might consider some type of volunteer role, so no need to continue to push on with my premorbid job. I later nicknamed such a forlorn situation when I would feel so broken "The Bleakness."

The Bleakness could be triggered by ubiquitous happy moments of everyday life. I was hypersensitive to common-day events that might cause a relapse. A child running happily around their parents, a couple walking hand and hand in the park and a commuting cyclist on the road felt like daggers to my heart as they reminded me of what I had lost. In an attempt to reach some measure of peace, I bargained with myself that I would give up such happy moments of life if I could just grasp some sense of normality.

Although there was such a merry life within touching distance just outside my window, I felt extremely distant from that. Instead, it was as far away as the moon. In the many instances when I found myself in such a despondent state, I would often find myself brooding. As I was later to find out, ruminating reactivates the pathways in your brain, making you re-live the event. Just thinking about the crash made me replay the "what ifs" again and again in my head. Yet although I attempted to escape The Bleakness, it seemed rather futile as my actions were thwarted at every turn. Too many things could trigger it and it simply wouldn't go away. When I thought that I had finally put it to bed, it would soon remind me that it was not dead with its unceasing tug and infinite patience. Sometimes it made me feel that trying to escape gravity would be more fruitful.

The Bleakness not only epitomised hopelessness but also a lack of direction and purpose. It sapped away my will to live as I struggled against a feeling that life wasn't worth living. I felt that I didn't have anything to reach for. No goals to achieve. No one to impress. With such melancholy thoughts overwhelming me, I felt that everything was so very pointless. If the world wouldn't notice if I was gone, why should I bother fighting? It would be easier to just give up.

On yet another day when I was again left alone in my hospital room, with my electric bed, drip cradle, panic cords and no one around, I came to realise something which I had been too wrapped up in my own troubles to realise. As life continued to pass by unconcerned with my anguish, I realised that few would even notice what I was going through, as it was all in my head. Even if they did, they wouldn't be able to help me. I would have to help myself.

In my search for a solution, I discovered that one particular emotion could provide something to blot out The Bleakness and give me direction. Anger could give me purpose. It provided something else to focus my thoughts on. Even though it was not healthy, it was much more preferable to vapid disinterest with the world. I found that feeling angry did not leave much space for aimlessness or sadness. As an additional benefit, feeling angry also satisfied my almost masochistic need to feel self-pity. I thought that of all people I had a right to be a very angry man and woe to anyone who thought to tell me otherwise. So this is how I came to cherish my anger. I cradled it lovingly for many months, as I felt that it gave me something to live for.

Yet I should have foreseen that it would not be without its own costs. Others around me with infinitely more wisdom could see that my anger was eating away at me. I ignored these people when they tried to counsel that I was sabotaging myself by not letting go. I found it very difficult to listen to such advice as I could not see how others had the right to tell me how to live my life. More poisonous still was when others might say "I know how you are feeling." Actually, I thought, they couldn't. They could take their advice and prattle it to someone else who was more able to escape their lecture. They shouldn't take advantage of my reduced circumstances and say such things to a hospital patient.

As time passed I became something of a connoisseur of rage. As I spent more time as an angry man, I found out an interesting fact – there were subtle nuances to anger. It was not simply a furnace of uniform heat but ranged from towering infernos to small pilot lights. What was manageable one day might be uncontainable another, and the danger was that no one could know what might light the kindling leading to an apocalyptic meltdown.

One thing that was almost guaranteed to cause an explosion was the mention of fault and blame. As I tried to change my view of blame, I wrestled to change my way of thinking that it was the fault of earthly and otherworldly beings that led to the position I was in. Perhaps it was just an extremely unfortunate series of events. After such exhausting sparring inside my head, I realised that I should instead just concentrate on the future. It would be counterproductive to dwell on finger-pointing and blame.

Yet even after settling all of this, I was still subject to a wild seesaw of emotions. Although I had managed to let go of thoughts of a possible divine attribution to my situation, the earthly attribution was another matter. I thought that if it was the fault of things in this world, then I was right to feel angry. Indeed, anger might even drive me to change my circumstances and make me better. Thankfully in time this phase passed and I returned to my quest to let go. As I struggled to let go of my anger, on my better days I tried to approach it through logic. I tried to convince myself that it was not useful and instead a waste of energy to live shackled to my anger. I simply couldn't live my life with a millstone around my neck. The anger would slowly wear away at me and whatever might be left would be an ugly and misshapen gnome.

Once I had resolved to deal with this anger, the next step was to try and release it. My initial method of dealing with my bitterness was to attempt to aggressively shove such unconstructive angry thoughts away into a little black box in the back of my mind. I would let the gremlins chew on them while I got on with life. This was easier said than done. At first it seemed like it wasn't working as the rock was too big and the hole in my box too small. Yet through my constant worrying about the hole, the edges slowly wore away and enlarged. Eventually I managed to pop most of the anger away and was able to mostly detach myself from this unhelpful emotion. Yet I still couldn't let go of the final strand as competing against this need to let go was my belief that I was entitled to be angry. I was also worried that if I let go of my anger, I might fall back into The Bleakness, so trading one demon for another.

In order to find another way to let go of this final part of anger, I had to try and find a different way to deal with The Bleakness. I came to realise that perhaps it would be helpful to re-characterise The Bleakness. Accordingly, I incrementally began to change my point of view to believe that traumatic brain injury was not the end of my life as I knew it. Instead, I should view it as a new beginning, a chance to rewrite my life. I tried to change my perspective by believing that although one door had shut, maybe another one had opened. It was just up to me to step through and seize the chance of a new life.

Reframing my perspective was the final step in my struggle to exile The Bleakness to its little box ready to be jettisoned. Once I had managed to pack away most of the remaining strands of this desolate and empty emotion, I discovered a welcome side effect. As I no longer had to hold on to anger to ward away The Bleakness, most of it faded away. In the absence of most of this burning emotion, I was then able to turn my attention to more productive matters – changing my perspective. To further assist with viewing things from a different point of view, I decided that writing would drive the final nail into the coffin of The Bleakness and I would be able to bury it. Putting my thoughts down on paper would stop the endless cycle. It was also hard to become angry at words on paper. Words wouldn't argue, attack or attempt to change me.

Yet I found that at this stage of my recovery, although writing would have been the ideal way to deal with The Bleakness, meaningful prose was unfortunately a little beyond my grasp as I was still having trouble dealing with my feelings. So to aid with putting The Bleakness behind me and also instil better emotional control, I instead resolved that it would be best to act like a mature, logical adult. Considered reasoning would be my way out and so with this goal in mind, I pondered how best to achieve this. Thankfully, a way seemed to almost drop into my lap as it overlapped with other issues that those around me were trying to resolve. I would need to not only think like a man but dress like one too.

Clothes make the man

Even though I had managed to overcome The Bleakness, this did not mean that it was all then smooth sailing. Once I had managed to escape the wheelchair, after a brief moment of euphoria, my resultant indifferent approach to life soon returned. At this stage, trying to cajole me into caring about myself was hopeless. I felt that there was little to live for as hospital felt like a prison, so why should I bother trying to get better? The crushing weight of my own hopes and dreams had all come crashing down into a million pieces and I felt that there wasn't any point in trying to put Humpty Dumpty back together again. This was especially true in the depressing locale of the hospital. It was so bad that I even had someone appointed to guard me 24/7, an orderly to ensure I wouldn't escape, rip essential tubes out of my body or engage in other foolhardy pursuits. Although he was there to look after me, I felt that his constant searching eyes were cataloguing everything I did so that he could report me if I stepped out of line with the facility's unwritten rules. I was too big now for a spanking, so stern words and guilt-tripping would be needed as an alternative.

When the staff saw me sinking further into this morose state, they tried their best to pull me out of it. Trying to shake me out of my uncaring state, the staff tried many different techniques. At first, the staff tried to treat me as though I were a baby. Babies did not have to worry about putting food on the table, looking after others or where the clothes on their back came from. Their world was much simpler to understand without such decisions to make. By removing my need for choice, they thought that I would be happier, yet this would not be the case. In fact, what I found most insulting was an attempt by the nursing staff to provoke a reaction by treating me like a small child at feeding time. An excerpt of some of the nurses' conversations with me follows: "Hello! Mr. Christopher! How are you today? Look at this lovely food we have today. Come on, open your mouth. Here comes the aeroplane …" I felt I had to remind some people that my crash did not mean I was now five.

These gentle and sometimes less so attempts to nudge me out of my uncaring state were often received in a glacial manner. Yet through unceasing prodding, I was eventually nudged out of my indifferent state. However, another problem then arose as in my new responsive state I found unceasing opportunities to complain. Viewing things from a different perspective though, the start of my moaning was actually a cause for celebration. It showed that I had been jolted out of my disinterest in life. Once I began to engage in mundane tasks, such as complaining about food, other concerns could be addressed as I now displayed some interest in the world.

Progressing on from this, the next stage was to try and instil in me some degree of attention to my appearance. Sometimes to the annoyance of others, my premorbid self had been slightly fastidious in dressing. At the start of the day, one little joy for him would be choosing what to wear for work. He would take care to dress in understated elegance, but now that choice had been taken away.

Starting in university, I had always been slightly fussy about how I dressed. Although I was limited by monetary policy and a need for multipurpose attire at that time, I could still dream. During my university years, I remember looking with envy at the smartly dressed gentlemen that passed me on the street. As my university was located near the Royal Courts of Justice, spiffy gentlemen were in abundance. I hoped that one day I would enter their esteemed company, with my own bespoke suit and a confident swagger. Then I would be the one that others would aspire to be, although I hoped that it would be without the seemingly dismissive, slightly arrogant manner.

Now in hospital, attire was chosen according to strictly proscribed limits. At the start I had no choice, as I was required to dress according to the occasion. Hospital dress is a very dehumanising experience for someone whose usual daily attire was a suit. I was instead relegated to a hospital gown. This opened at the back, giving easy access to my rear receptacles. It also made it easy to accidently flash people. As an additional complication when I was wheelchair bound, not being able to walk to the toilet also made for interesting sanitary arrangements. To deal with this problem, I was to become well acquainted with a wheelchair with a convenient hole in the middle – a toilet on wheels. Termed a commode, this would prove to be a piece of equipment I grew to loathe. Said item would also serve a dual purpose as a shower. Although at least this was a step up from having my urinary processes managed by catheters.

Fortunately, being in a private hospital, I was encouraged to take charge of my dressing as soon as possible. I was encouraged to wear my own clothes and paper pyjamas were to be reverted to only when strictly required, such as during more invasive procedures. As was no doubt the intention, the ability to select my clothes played a key part in my journey to regain my dignity. It was easier to be taken seriously without the rustle of paper every time I moved. The restoration of my attire, although it was rather ill-fitting in my case as a result of my loss of fifteen kilograms in weight, produced a corresponding lift in my mood. It shifted my self-perception from being an invalid needing to be helped with basic functions and began the long journey back to ordinary human life, something which I had regarded with disdain before but now eagerly awaited. Boring and ordinary activities took on a new shine. I dreamt of being able to go to the supermarket to shop for dinner.

Having relived at least the first part of the cradle to the grave journey in full, excruciating detail, I became very sensitive to what others thought of me. Did the T-shirt fit my style of hair? Did the socks match the shirt? Were my shoes appropriate? I admit I became even more obsessive and fastidious in my dressing habits following my accident. I felt that how I dressed was very important as it was an element that I could influence relatively easily. It was my way to control people's perceptions of me without saying a word. As an added benefit, it would provide further distraction from any other issues I might display. Being so carefully dressed, I found it was much easier to convince people that I was an articulate and bright young man. I tried to present myself well so people would not feel any need to dig into my past.

On the flip side, the dress of other people was also an important point. With my cognition processes so compromised at the start of my recovery, visual cues from how people dressed were important, not only to avoid embarrassment but merely to be able to live a normal life. At the start of my recovery due to my severe memory deficits, I would often not be able to remember people, even though they introduced themselves again and again for days. For example, the physiotherapist who treated me daily for three weeks in my critical period is sadly a blur. With such a problem, daily introductions of who people were had to be repeated day after day, as I explained in brief in "The Wellington hospital."

These constant reintroductions also depleted my very limited store of cognitive energy, as although I could make some small talk on the surface with no recollection of who I was talking to, underneath I would be frantically struggling to figure out who it was in front of me. To reduce the load on my brain, I tried to find hints and shortcuts to live my life. One such way was using first impressions to conserve my brain power as I would guess based on what people wore. The person dressed in light blue scrubs must be a surgeon. The person dressed in a suit must be a doctor. However, visual cues can be misleading. I could easily be confused if the clothing was reversed. To someone like me in a state of cognitive agitation, I may very well have thought that a doctor dressed as a clown was a clown.

For such reasons, the uniforms worn at the hospital were very helpful. They reduced the cognitive load much in the same way that the various signs around the hospital helpfully pointed out directions to various rooms. I didn't have to keep maps in my head; there was already a queue for the scarce mental real estate. Instead, using other people's dress as clues, I could be confident enough of whom I was rolling and later walking with to ask questions or plead for help. It wouldn't do if I asked a janitor for help with a neuropsychological issue. I idly wondered if it worked the other way as well. Did the nurses identify the patients by their dress or lack thereof? Would they have difficulty identifying me if I wasn't in my usual hospital attire? If I dressed in eye-wateringly bright clothes with flowers in my hair, would I be taken to be over the moon or maybe just a bit loony?

Thankfully I was spared having to muddle my way through such a situation. By the time of my discharge I was dressing "normally," although this was mainly due to the help of my family who would pick out what I was to wear and cajole me when I was a bit reluctant to dress appropriately. Sometimes when I argued with family when I refused to take care of my appearance, I was keen to stress to them that hospital dress had another benefit. If I wore it, I wouldn't have to make the effort to decide anything. I would be able to ration my mental energy for more important things. Although they gently reminded me that presenting well was part of normal life, so they would not be discouraged in their nagging.

Although my selection and interest in attire paled in comparison to other problems I had, the constant prodding eventually had its desired effect. I began to care about my dress and, as no doubt was the intention, this had unexpected benefits. By the end of this line of treatment, I was dressing a bit more ordinarily and my outlook on life seemed to brighten with my interest in and freedom to choose how I dressed. Clothes did indeed make the man, but now that I had begun to pay attention to my attire, I could move onto the next step: learning to act my age.

A birthday in hospital

Looking back, I wonder if I should have dressed up for my birthday. Yet even if I had access to an unlimited wardrobe, I doubt I would have been in the mood. For me, birthdays are not events that I celebrate with pomp and circumstance, as I usually do not particularly note or await them with uncontainable anticipation. I found that as I grew older, they began to lose their significance. When I was turning five, it was the most important event in the whole wide world. When I turned twenty-five, it was just another mark to be added to the scratch card. This apathy was particularly memorable once when I was in university, when I forgot that a particular day was my birthday. I only noticed when I had to fill out that particular day's date on a job application form. Imagine my surprise when the dates seemed to match! I found it a bit amusing that I had stumbled across such a discovery at four p.m. in the anticlimactic and frantic environment of the university library, in a locale filled with students desperately studying or purveying the classified ads. I then quickly found it sad that I found such a situation funny.

My birthday in the year of my incident was to be a particularly memorable departure from the norm. I went to sleep in my hospital bed the night before my birthday, fervently wishing that this was all a bad dream. I thought that if I wished hard enough, when I woke up, the hospital would be no more. That would be a most excellent birthday gift. Alas, life conspired to continue to make my life "interesting." When I woke up again on my birthday in the same grey hospital room, I first looked around in sad expectation hoping to find that something had changed. I stared at the cupboard and wished that someone would burst out and tell me that I had been part of some colossal joke, but this was slightly delusional thinking. With cheery events failing to materialise, I felt in desperate need of something to lift my spirits. After the realisation of my situation had sunk in again, and I realised that the callous reality would not be changing, I desperately tried to find a silver lining to counterbalance my disappointment. What I finally settled on as a positive (if you can call it that) was that I should feel "honoured" to experience something few others would, a birthday in hospital. That would be something to tell if I was ever asked to share an unusual experience.

Once the hospital did not magically disappear, I began to harbour hidden hopes that I would get to do something special as a consolation prize for coming to terms with the harsh, unwelcome truth. Later that morning, it seemed that such a wish might come true when my occupational therapy for the day was announced; I was ecstatic, as it was something unusual. I would make a rare out-of-hospital excursion to a pre-arranged destination by myself. I thought in my excitement that maybe this was my birthday present; to be let out of the hospital unsupervised. At this stage I truly treasured opportunities to mingle with the crowd.

However, the real reason for this special excursion was to assess whether I would display signs of confusion and/or anxiety attacks on my solo trip. The concern was that as these are common following a severe knock to the head, they might pertain to me too. Although I thought that once I stepped out of the hospital on my errand that I was unsupervised, I was later to find out that I had been secretly shadowed the whole time, in case I panicked, got lost, started to consume various plastic objects or all of the above. Fortunately, I was recovered enough that I did not engage in such antisocial behaviour.

After mingling in the wider public, once my city tasks were complete, I arrived at the pre-agreed final destination. Here I met my therapist and sought further instructions. She then asked me to find my own way back to the hospital. Confusion followed as I was barred from asking others for assistance. A rather comical scene then played out. This was of me trying to locate and interpret the various maps around the station and orientate myself indoors. This exercise was fairly fruitless, but I was rescued when my attempts attracted the attention of nearby station staff who helpfully pointed me in the direction of the bus station. Nothing had been said about refusing the unsolicited help of others. Having almost completed a job well done, my therapist then asked me what the time was to see if I was keeping track of the clock. It was at this opportunity that I presented my wrist, with wristband and watch.

Here it might be helpful if I gave a bit of context about my wristband. Upon admission, all Wellington hospital, patients are tagged so that the staff can easily identify them. The band displays vitals such as name, blood type, ward and date of birth. When I first arrived, I had one on each ankle and one around each wrist. Made out of plastic, they are water and rip-proof (believe me I tried). The number and location of these was to prevent mixing up or misplacing patients and the idea was that although you might gnaw the band off your wrist, the ankle would prove more difficult unless you were unusually flexible. I soon grew to hate these manacles, which shouted to the world at large that I was "special." I was irritated at times as I felt that I was being treated as a lab rat, tagged for easy assessment of experimental treatment. No, I would not like to be irradiated again. No, I don't see how it would help me. No, why don't you do it yourself if you want to glow in the dark. Happily for me, the quantity of these restraining devices was reduced as I became more independent, finally settling on an indivisible number, just one around my left wrist.

Returning here to my name day celebration, once I had presented my watch including adjacent wristband to the therapist, I then pointed at my watch and said that we had plenty of time to return to the hospital. My watch also displayed the day, which was now adjacent to the date on my wristband. The therapist's reaction was gratifying, as she realised that today was my birthday. I quipped when she seemed speechless, was it because I was more mature than her? She was not amused as it was true. At this stage, I made no comment because I thought that might undermine the perception of mental maturity I was particularly keen to demonstrate.

Once I got off the bus and returned to hospital, I was deposited back in my room. After a short amount of time, my family arrived to attempt to cheer me up with a birthday cake which had been waiting in the hospital patiently (if a cake can wait patiently for its own demise). I knew that the socially correct action for me to take was to exclaim about the generosity of others. I duly marvelled at the cake and exclaimed, "How did you know I liked chocolate cake?" I then ate a slice of it to be polite, but the truth was that to me, it tasted of opportunities lost.

A massive argument then erupted with my family. I cannot remember the details but from what I can recall, it was because I felt much self-pity. In such a mood, I felt that attempts to cheer me up were full of so much false cheer. It only served to remind me of what ifs. This accordingly made me flick between quicksilver bouts of despondency and rage. I felt that people shouldn't pretend that things were alright and that a birthday in hospital was still an event to be celebrated. I found it almost inexcusable that they had not bothered to discuss how I would like my birthday in hospital to go. If they had, they would understand what their actions were doing. If they couldn't make the hospital magically disappear, I did not want to be reminded of my birthday. In such a state I unfairly became very angry at my family caringly trying to put on a brave happy face. It came to such a head that I stormed off into the rain, not to cool off my hot head but in search of suffering to match my mood.

Fortunately for me, I was chased down by my father who was very concerned that I might catch a cold and create further complications in the cold pouring rain. With the benefit of hindsight, it is now clear to me that this was another sign of my childish mental capacity and unwillingness to face reality. At that time I wanted to get sick out of some masochistic sense that I needed physical pain to match my mental anguish. To that end, I thought that it was very fitting that on such a bleak, cold, wet and miserable day, I would spend what was supposed to be one of the happiest days of my life in hospital. I thought that I could now chalk up another episode to a life lived by contrast.

In the end my father managed to persuade me to return to the Wellington hospital, but here I had yet another surprise. The hospital staff unwittingly made a surprise appearance to wish me happy birthday, which was a touching gesture. I guess due to the nature of their job they have little occasion to celebrate. What they did not know was that I had had a small meltdown in the pouring rain. Unaware and oblivious to the situation, their genuine cheer and happiness in celebrating my birthday burnt like hot coals on my heart. The more gusto that people around me conjured in celebration, the deeper the wound as all I could hear were the shards of shattered dreams drifting mournfully by.

Although my emotional age was quite juvenile as shown by my recent actions, I still retained enough sense to know that the best way to convince everyone to go away would be to put on a face of false cheer, no matter how brittle. Although I doubt that my family was fooled, they eventually left me alone as they understood that they could do nothing further and that I needed some time alone. I was growing impatient to return to my solo life as I felt that I needed to have some solitude to sulk and I couldn't do this with other people watching. Amongst such surroundings, I spent one of my birthdays in the prime of my life in hospital. It was, to use a British euphemism, "interesting." Even more so, in a head trauma unit with the "exciting" background noises of groaning, ranting and occasionally screaming, this was not a day to quickly forget.

So this is how I found myself sitting in my hospital room by myself and thinking about where I had dreamed and planned to be on this day. On my adventure of a lifetime, discovering the meaning of my life, making new lifelong friends and settling my career track for the next couple of years. Instead, in this literally and figuratively sterile world, I sat down and moped for paradise lost.

A tilted point of view

If I could have had any birthday wish in the world granted, I would have wished for my normal sight back. As a result of the incident, I see two of everything. It leads to an interesting life.

It is maybe good for some things, like cake (I must have been a good boy because I now see two), but not so good for things like the stairs (where did that extra stair that tripped me up come from?). To try and mitigate the effects, I wore a patch over one eye to prevent my confusion. This solved one problem but considering the exciting way that my life was, I should have expected that it would throw up something new.

In my pirate mode, I also suffered from another ancillary issue, I lacked stereo vision. As a consequence of only having one eye, I saw the world in two dimensions. I wasn't able to see depth and literally could not grasp the point. As a result of my flat perception, I would often grasp at air as I could not tell where objects were in space. Yet this meant that my life was easier to understand as there was less to understand in a two-dimensional world – the flat world was more straightforward and easier to comprehend. Things just didn't seem to have depth so I did not have to spend time puzzling out if there was more to things. Life was instead rather shallow and easier to understand. In the first year post incident, I would not be bothered with less important externalities, as simple was good.

Although this lack of perception helped me to live an uncomplicated life, it also caused entirely foreseeable problems. Living in a three-dimensional world while only able to perceive its flat nature was a physical manifestation of my stunted mental state. This led to a couple of uncomfortable and occasionally painful situations as I lacked comprehension of how reality worked. In particular, I could not understand why my invalidity was not accorded with due respect. I had initially hoped that with a patch over my eye, people would take a bit more care around me. I was to be sorely disappointed in this respect.

The outside world treated me by and large with a lack of compassion. This was even more so than when I was in a wheelchair. Although on occasion people would give me a bit more space, most of the time I would have to be on my guard as they might simply barge into me, maybe in the hopes that I was like a *piñata* and would drop sweets if hit hard enough. My anger at such instances would grow and grow and, on such occasions, I would often stare at people's backs and await divine intervention. Unfortunately, such supernatural retribution has to my knowledge failed to be delivered. Although, unlike my wheelchair days, I could console myself with the knowledge that I could follow them and rain verbal abuse if I so wished.

Yet I soon learned that although I could simmer and await otherworldly punishment, it wouldn't help me in the here and now. As a reoccurring theme of my recovery, although I felt angry at my situation, the constructive thing was just to move on. Struggling out of The Bleakness taught me that there was no point crying over spilt milk. So to cope with this flat world, I had to figure out a way to survive. I found that the most efficient way to live my life in this way was to develop hyperawareness of what others were doing. Through this I learnt about the world from the perspective of others.

Again, I thought that this had many similarities to being a child, learning about the world by watching how others interacted in it. It was almost a case of monkey see, monkey do. Through this process of living relatively, I could discover that the series of lines on the floor were actually stairs after people slowed to mount them. The surrounding people would give me clues as to the lay of the land. I would be warned of potential dangers by the pausing of fellow pedestrians. I could learn to cross the road by watching others. Life could be lived relatively.

I thought that this was not so different from the way I lived pre-incident, as I was always consciously or unconsciously influenced by the people around me, although not in such an obvious physical way. The real difference now was that my physical well-being would be an issue when there was no one else around. Using others as stalking horses was all well and good, but when they had all bolted, things were a bit difficult. In lonely moments, with no one there to be the unwitting guinea pig, I would need to feel my way through life's events with a stick.

So with this lack of spatial awareness, I had to learn what was underneath the simple world. I had thought that I would have no problem understanding what things were with a shift in viewpoint, but what I discovered was that losing one axis of visual perception could make all the difference. The familiar could become very alien with a tilted point of view.

Things were so different from learning about what things were for the first time as building my understanding of what things were again was a rather bitter process. Instead of the bright-eyed wonder and ecstatic fascination with the discovery of new objects that I might have shown as a child, as an invalid seeing things for the second time, there was instead resignation and poignancy that I hadn't managed to figure out what things were sooner. Rediscovery felt like chewing ashes as in such situations I would feel that I had let myself down.

When I was caught with such melancholy thoughts running through my mind, I would then wonder if perhaps my life was a particularly twisted type of TV show. As I couldn't judge depth, life had to be lived with abundant caution. The little spire could be a model or the real thing in the distance, other pedestrians could be closer than I thought, the circle on the pavement could be a drawing or a hole waiting to swallow me up. I just couldn't know.

In more dangerous situations, this posed particular issues when crossing the road. I couldn't see how far away cars were, which caused unnecessary excitement when living in the city. In a similar way to dealing with stairs, I tried to conquer this obstacle by watching other people. In such a way, I could use them to help judge when it was safe for me to cross the road. However, I was soon to find out that this was not by any means risk free. If the person I was watching was careless, lacking in awareness or not particularly nimble, I might be an unwitting lemming coming to play in the traffic.

Removing the ability to see from one eye had an interesting side effect; in medical terminology, it is known as right side spatial neglect. Not only did I see the world in two dimensions, but I lost comprehension of one side. At first this seemed nonsensical, as even babies would realise that if you played peek-a-boo, half of the world did not disappear when you covered one of their eyes. Yet proof of the validity of how this condition affected me was shown by the significant amount of accidents I had on my blind side. I would constantly walk into things on my right, swiping cups and stationary off tables, not noticing people standing on that side and in one notable instance, walking straight into a lamp post. As the consequences generally increased in severity related to mass, I realised that to avoid another visit to the hospital, I would have to be more careful. I would accordingly try to give extra space on my blind side. As I later learned, the reason for this rather interesting side effect was that if you have one eye covered, your very ability to perceive that side slowly disappears. It is as if you cannot comprehend that there is a second half to your body. It is as if the brain turns off its proprioception and sees you as a half man.

To make things more interesting, this slightly skewed view was combined with another issue; not only did I see two cakes, but one cake appeared to be happily sliding up the wall. As a result of this, I was reprimanded gently by one of my therapists as I was often tilting my head to compensate for this. When I tilted my head in a certain way, the world came back into single focus. I fervently wished that my other problems could be dealt with by such a simple manoeuvre, but I was unfortunately not living in a fairy tale.

This slightly unusual requirement to help put things back on a level footing led to a rather interesting sight, a young man who appeared to have his head permanently bent at an angle. When I saw pictures of myself, it seemed that I was perpetually listening to a song that no one else could hear. That was not that far from the truth, as sometimes it felt like I was listening to the unending litany in my head of has-beens and worries about days to come.

Yet several months later, once my eye condition had stabilised, I was surprised with unexpected hope when one of my doctors mentioned that there might be a quick surgical fix for my tilted point of view. I could hardly contain my excitement and dreamt of things coming back into normal focus. I found myself very much looking forward to going under the scalpel again and counted the scars on my body, preparing for one more.

Yet after the operation when the bandages came off, and after I had impatiently waited a couple of days, things did not revert back to normal. A risk that the surgeon had previously tried to warn me was a likely possibility had materialised: the correction was not complete and things might never look normal again. In my blind hope, I had glazed over and ignored such a warning and the danger was that further tinkering might make the problem worse. Although initially rather disappointed, I slowly learnt to come to terms with this different point of view. As the doctor later remarked in a follow-up appointment, if I was completely fixed, life would be kind of boring and he jokingly said he wouldn't want that.

Learning to adapt to my slanted perspective, I now walk around with a more upright bearing, with my head held high and straight. Shifting my view to instead look on the brighter side of things, I told myself that my tilted view could be a constant reminder to carefully consider different perspectives in everything I did or saw. It would be a gentle admonition that I should not judge things so hastily. It was perhaps fitting that it should happen to me in my particular set of circumstances; brain injury was not easily perceived as damage was hidden where the eye could not see.

As the days went by and as I got used to my tilted point of view, half the time I managed to convince myself that things were actually not that bad. Learning some lessons from my other injuries, I tried to approach this problem with a more adult frame of mind and just get used to things if I couldn't change them. It would seem rather childish to practise some wilful blindness, especially so soon after my birthday, and so I tried to tell myself that this problem was relatively minor. There were much bigger problems to tackle than sight. What was the use of perfect vision if I didn't have a self to appreciate it?

The assault on self

Try as I might to shut my eyes to my reduced circumstances, this rather childish behaviour was rarely effective and was my attempt to ignore the core of my grief, the diminishing of my mental prowess. My crash made me feel as though my brain was assaulted in some dark alley and I had been mugged of something core to my being. Ignorance was not bliss as I found that my troubles would not go away if I just left them to ferment. Many of the issues with my changed self sprung from this refusal to accept my new self.

In my struggle to conceptualise this damage to others, I would explain that my crash caused such a change from my status quo that it was like I had to rewrite my concept of self. Resorting to metaphors and imagery, I would explain that it felt to me as brutal as a shot to the head. Sometimes it would feel that I had had half of my brain blown out by a blunderbuss. Yet try as I might to convey this to others, it was rarely effective. I did wonder if this lack of understanding by others was because I didn't show any obvious infirmities. Maybe if I hobbled around with a stick they might show more empathy. Following my crash, I felt that I was a lesser man. It seemed terribly unfair that all the hardship and suffering I had to endure to reach my pedestal of premorbid life was all wiped away in an instant by the crash.

If someone had asked me what my greatest vanity was, I would have replied that it was my intellect. I treasured it so dearly, it being all that was really me. Now I would have the "excitement" of having it undermined. For others, the core of what they are is their physical prowess. James Cracknell has also spoken about this in his book *Touching Distance* (2013), where he suffered a severe brain injury while riding a bicycle. Ironically his incident was on the same day of the year as mine. Maybe that date is somehow cursed for cyclists. He also ended up in the same hospital as me, the Wellington hospital. Thankfully his story is one filled with hope as with the support of his wife, he went on to make an excellent recovery. In fact, he provides motivational speeches to this day. I could only push on in the hope that I might attain some measure of his success.

Although James achieved an "against all odds recovery," I would hazard a guess that he still feels like all brain injury survivors, that something is different about the world now. Even though I was able to recover physically relatively rapidly, my mental healing was markedly slower. I also felt that damage to my mental faculties was so much more devastating than the physical infirmities because it could not be seen by outsiders. As people could not see my difficulties, they would not think to lend me a helping hand. This was in contrast to more physical injuries, such as a broken arm or leg, which were more readily apparent to others around me. With more visible injuries such as these, people would usually give up their seat on a crowded tube. Yet with a mental injury, by its very nature being inside my head, it did not allow for easy recognition. This troubled me as sometimes in the early days of my recovery I could see the unspoken question in people's eyes when they met me doing something atypical on the street: why was I acting somewhat "funny"?

My own recognition of my temporarily reduced mental capacity was also difficult for me personally to comprehend and accept. It was demonstrated to me by atypical scores in various tests I took when compared to the expected results based on my educational and occupational history. These examinations took place over months and were so numerous that they seemed to blur together. Yet one in particular that stuck in my mind was the digit span test to examine my working memory. In this examination, I was read a series of numbers and was then asked to repeat them back. A comparison was made against the national average, seven. I scored four. This was blindly obvious to me now as I was having trouble remembering the start of my conversations at times. Yet at that time, it was very unwelcome news and depression soon set in. Trying to lift my spirits, the doctors and therapists were keen to stress that even months after my crash, these were still the early days of recovery. Yet with these results, I felt that my times of doing complicated equations were well and truly gone. I couldn't even remember a couple of simple numbers. With such issues, how could I even think about doing quadratic equations or even simply adding up the grocery bill in my head?

Realising that such results depressed me mightily, my family tried to show me that life really wasn't all that bad. So sometime into my recovery, my doctors deemed that I could handle some small degree of additional stimulation. My family then accordingly allowed visitors into my hospital room once I was well enough to carry on contrived conversations. The idea was that my positive feelings would be bolstered by meeting people outside of my then limited circle.

Through this process, I came to understand how valuable friendships were when you were down. In particular, I owe particular debts of gratitude to friends who helped in their own special ways. One was an old friend who I hadn't really kept in contact with but would do almost anything for me. I later found out that he was more than ready to drop everything to fly out to be at my side while I was in a remote French hospital. Another provided true emphatic discussion as he could truly say that he did know how I felt having suffered a severe smack to the head himself. As we sat down one day and he explained his experiences, I found it immensely helpful to see how he had overcome them. Yet other assistance came in the form of an unlikely but touching gesture. One friend turned up one day to my hospital room clutching a flask of special herbal soup. I thought this was particularly thoughtful as she could not really cook. Maybe the best place to taste her food was in hospital, where easy and speedy access to emergency equipment would be readily available if anything went awry.

Yet such visits did not always go as planned. Even if they were appreciated, they were sometimes stunted as depending on my mood I could be a less than willing participant. When I was in a melancholy mood, at times I simply could not care less that some people had dropped by and I would be rather taciturn. In such a situation, trying to prompt me out of my unresponsive state, my visitors would ask me where I would want to go for a holiday, where I wished to visit when I was out of hospital and what I dreamed of eating for dinner. I would often give some extremely vague response or would simply not answer as I felt that such things were so far away and not even something I would contemplate in my misery. I just felt that there was nothing left inside myself and such dreams of normality were grossly unrealistic.

I felt that my past self had been cruelly severed by the crash and the future me was too crippled to care. This prompted a particular type of response when I was feeling especially listless. On such occasions when the questioning became too much I would respond with emptiness. I just couldn't summon the requisite enthusiasm to make small talk. Instead, I would just let people see what I felt inside. In such situations, I just wanted to be left alone. As a side benefit, sometimes this type of response would scare people off.

While in such a pensive mood, when others were bothering me so, the screaming unfairness of the world was more apparent. I found that the saying the taller they are, the harder they fall is very accurate. I found that I couldn't always trust myself as sometimes I just did not make sense. When this was brought to my attention by people I trusted, my then fragile confidence was shattered. This inability to trust myself would constantly undermine me, and for someone who had been quite sure of himself, doubt was a terrifying alien. Although I might have been confident in decisions I made, such certainty was rare. Even when it was present, it would not linger long and would quickly flee.

In the early days of my recovery, when I made a decision, I would question myself as others would remind me time and time again that my judgement was suspect. What made this even more hurtful was that sometimes other people would use this fact to their advantage. When it was with concern, I could understand. When it was with the intention of manipulation, I became an angry man, especially when people decided to play the ultimate trump card, "you don't know better." What made that seemingly normal blow in an argument a gut punch was the scary thought that they might be right.

Through such experiences, I became suspicious of almost everyone. I would constantly be on my guard as it seemed that everyone had their own agenda and it might not be in my best interests. Sensing this sceptical and mistrustful attitude, one day one of my doctors pulled me aside. He tried to reassure me that I was not crazy and that he was on my side. He was keen to stress that his duty of care was only to me. In essence, he was alluding to the fact that I could at any moment tell everyone to go away. Although many people around me would have had a vested interest in my recovery, it might be somewhat influenced by their own motivation. Instead, my doctor pointed out that he only had a duty to me as I was in his charge. I might be damaged but I was still my own man. He was a doctor to me only, not my parents, my friends or the random visitors. It was my life to succeed or fail in and I quite rightly should be in the driving seat.

It was after one particular discussion with my medical team and family that things came to a head. It was at this point that I had vehemently disagreed with the wishes of my family, who wanted things one way, and my medical team, who were of a differing opinion. Following this, my doctor pointed out to my family and I that this substantial disagreement and my subsequent reasoned refusal to cave was a sign that I could now make my own decisions. Other people could say all they wanted, but I would be the one that would need to actually live with the outcome. If I felt strongly one way and had thought about it carefully, it was my prerogative to choose how to proceed.

Although this experience was far from pleasant, through this I proved that the new me was able to fend for himself. I was now prepared to deal with conflict and face the consequences of my decisions. I would not need family or medical personnel to oversee my every action. I could handle arguments with people without falling apart. Although my acceptance of my new self was not complete at this point, it was sufficient. My doctors then considered it appropriate to progress to the next stage of my treatment. In life there would be many pitfalls and setbacks, but if I tripped and fell into a hole, I would survive – and at least it would be my hole.

End of an era

Many months after my crash and after I had finally come to some degree of acceptance about my changed self, the time came for discharge from the Wellington hospital. My time in hospital felt like an eternity and although the hospital staff had done their utmost to make my exercises challenging, it was now time for the real world, as I no longer suffered from any critical deficits. The time for practice was over and I had to bid goodbye to the simulations.

The concern was that I would need to practise real-world applications of my skills. The exercises in the hospital were mainly done under laboratory conditions and were therefore untested in actual situations. Although I was now pushed out into the real world, an immediate and jarring transition to a completely normal life might have been too much. The shock might kill me. As an intermediate step, I would embark on a staged discharge by attending the hospital as an outpatient every day. It would have the additional benefit of forcing me to accustom myself to commuting like millions of workers.

As the day for discharge drew closer, I grew more and more excited at leaving what I viewed at times as a hospice. Unlike university or high school, I could see little reason for any nostalgia when graduating from hospital, as it contained few happy memories. Although the most traumatic instances of my recovery were thankfully not remembered because of my amnesia, when I was ever in the locale, I couldn't shake a sense of foreboding about the Wellington hospital.

As it was later put to me, this was perhaps a very distorted way of seeing my incarceration in the hospital. I might be suffering from a great sense of entitlement as others would not have had as great an opportunity to recover. I should feel lucky that I was given one of the best chances to heal. When I was in a more contemplative mood, I had a niggling feeling that in the end the Wellington hospital was something to be thankful for, even despite some shaky moments. Although it was the centre of so much pain and suffering in my life, it was also the place where I learnt to walk, talk and pretend to function like a normal person. It provided a safety net while I was exploring the new me in an accommodating environment where failure was accepted. It was a place of rebirth.

Yet leaving the hospital did not mean that I would be out of the woods yet. Regular life would still be full of its own pitfalls and potential for failures. Foreseeing this danger, a large element of my latter days of treatment at the Wellington hospital concentrated on my ability to handle setbacks. In trying to build up my resilience, I was taught time and time again not to give up but to continue to press forward. I was encouraged to use my witty (others would say morbid or sarcastic) turn of phrase and sense of humour to lessen the blow, so when I inevitably fell I would still pick myself up. Another reason to rationalise discharge was that in the hospital the well-meaning hospital staff couldn't help but cushion the fall, in contrast to the rather harder concrete of the real world. Reality just did not have as much give. Outside the hospital there would be no panic button for me to push in times of need. No friendly medical staff to explain to me why I found life so difficult. No encouragement that things would eventually get better.

As the date for discharge drew closer, a mild degree of panic took hold of me. What would I do if I experienced a relapse? How would I deal with situations where I couldn't get my message across? What would happen if I couldn't cope? Why was I being let out so early, I wasn't ready! Such situations played endlessly through my mind. As I was becoming used to it, the end of my days in the hospital came with a lack of fanfare.

On the day of my discharge, I woke up in the morning to partake in my last hospital meal. After finishing my bread and butter, I packed up my meagre belongings and checked that nothing was left under the bed or behind the cupboard. I then sat down in my chair to wait for my check-out process. It was a vain hope that the hospital was immune to a large pile of paperwork. Welcome back to real life indeed. Eventually the matron arrived with various forms to complete. While I was filling out my details, she proceeded to undertake a final sweep of the room to check that I had not managed to fit the TV into my backpack.

Eventually she was satisfied with my paperwork and then left me alone. I finally had a moment by myself. With all my check-out formalities complete, I then got up to leave. As I walked out of my room, at the exit, I did pause at the door and take a look back. This was where I had spent a great deal of the most traumatic time of my life. I peered back to see the motorised hospital bed that I had spent so many sleepless nights in. The little table where I had started writing my story. The worn armchair where I had sat in my depressed state so many times. The balcony door that I had never been through.

This was a room of so much hurt, despair and anger, yet also hope, determination and sometimes peace. Turning around, I thought that it was time to close this chapter of my life. It would be best if I put "such bad things" behind me.

So I shut the door.

The National Health Service

Between the next scheduled major rehabilitation appointment at the Oliver Zangwill Centre, a specialist neurorehabilitation centre, and my discharge from the Wellington hospital, I had a bit of a break from my structured treatment regime. My family and I decided that the best way to fill this gap was with treatment at my local community hospital. With this eventuality in mind, before my discharge from the Wellington hospital, my treatment team had been in touch with local community services to ensure that I had all the support and treatment I would require. It seemed to be handled fully and correctly, as the National Health Service (NHS) health worker assigned to my case promised me the world. Although I was initially rather sceptical, I thought I needed to trust them. It wasn't like I had any other choice.

When I finally started treatment after being on the waiting list for quite some time, I admit to being in somewhat of a sour mood due to the delay. I had been put in line several months before my discharge, but only several weeks following my discharge was I at the front of the queue. My apprehension was also fed by various friends who worked as doctors. They portrayed a rather negative view of the NHS, maybe because they did not want me to get my hopes up. I should accordingly not expect to get any significant help from them. From such a low bar it would not be hard to be disappointed.

Starting my treatment, I tried to put aside my prejudices. I endeavoured to throw myself wholeheartedly into this new regime of treatment. Yet my old biases still managed to reassert themselves, even though I was determined to give the NHS the benefit of the doubt. It was a good thing that I hadn't written off the NHS but had given it a chance, as I was to find that the psychologist assigned to my case was particularly skilled. She had dealt with people exhibiting symptoms like me before and had much experience dealing with difficult patients. Although I arrived at our first meeting prepared to engage in a contest of wills, she managed to handily disarm me by showing that she held no prejudices.

Although I arrived at my first meeting ready for a fight, my psychologist blunted my assertiveness by showing that she did not have any preconceived notions of me. It was rather hard for me to hold on to my own prejudices in this light. I had come to my first meeting prepared with a long list of questions in my book, pen ready for battle, yet by the end of the meeting, I found flowing smooth handwriting instead of enraged scribbling on my paper. With the benefit of hindsight, what I determined was her secret to success was simple. She treated me as a person. Not a faceless number in a book. Not as another damaged statistic, but as someone fragile, weak and altogether human.

Unlike other therapists I had met, she was determined not to treat me as if I was a square person that would fit into a round hole. She was careful not to put my hackles up and instead was ready to genuinely listen. As I recounted my worries and troubles she would patiently take notes. She would make appropriate noises to show that she appreciated that I was a real person with my own thoughts, dreams and failings. Then, with carefully considered questions, when I despaired of continuing on she asked me to consider looking at things a different way.

In particular, she addressed my failure to be heard by the ones closest to me. I complained bitterly that my family did not seem to listen to me and disregarded my decision-making ability. With much patience she demonstrated that my decisions were still considered and rational based on the information provided. I wasn't some five-year-old trying to stubbornly insist on getting his way. Instead, I was a frustrated, fully fledged adult with grown-up problems. Through our many sessions, she repeated time and time again that I had been changed but it was up to me whether this would make me a better or worse person.

Moving on to other matters, she also tried to deal with my anger and depression. To do this she provided a sympathetic ear for me to voice how unhappy I was with the cruelty of the world. As she commiserated with me over things lost, I would like to think that during these sessions the constant nodding and words of compassion and agreement were genuine, but I slowly came to realise that the basis for such a consensus did not really matter. It was enough that someone would take my side after seemingly everyone tried to second-guess my decisions. That someone would sit down and really listen, even if it was just pretend listening, helped me to realise that I wasn't a bit unhinged. Through this treatment my psychologist assured me that my worries and troubles were no more than those of any other person on the street.

Once we had established that I wasn't crazy, widely erratic or schizophrenic, together we dug down into my psyche to discover what was underlying my self-torture. What we discussed was that it seemed like I was stuck in a no man's land. My old self was behind, punishing me with trophies of my past life. My new self was just ahead, waiting for an embrace. What she explained was that to put my old worries to bed, all I had to do was look forward. It was actually the height of folly to think that an event as traumatic as the crash would not change me. Instead I should focus my energies on moving forward.

Unfortunately, it was not all positive things in the NHS. Through this slow journey of discovery I did manage to learn one thing about the NHS: the excessive bureaucracy. To get just about anything done, it felt like forms had to be filled out in triplicates. At times it appeared that wringing blood out of a stone would have been easier than trying to get appropriate treatment.

My doctors, my family and I had been fighting for months for funding to attend the Oliver Zangwill Centre, itself another NHS centre. Although apparently it seemed that someone had decided that once I was walking and talking that was all that needed to be done. It was as though I didn't need anything else and I should be content just to reach their arbitrary level of recovery. This was despite medical advice from doctors stating in no uncertain terms what in their opinion would be best. Yet, things did not pan out this way. I should have known that paperwork could overcome even the most exemplary of us.

Regrettably in the NHS, it seemed that sometimes desirable treatment would fall through the gaps. Protection of the public purse could sometimes lead to suffering and ironically more pain for the tax payer. If people fell again, it was the NHS who would need to pick up the pieces. The eternal tug of war in the NHS caused much heartbreak and suffering at times, although this was balanced by the excellence of its treatment if you managed to get to the right place at the right time.

When I later managed to speak to other traumatic brain injury survivors, I heard many examples of stories of their attempts to seek treatment. One had been ignored for years and was thought of as stupid and lazy because he couldn't do things himself. In the end he just needed an understanding therapist to explain why he found things so difficult and to show him a way to overcome his problems. Another was just angry all the time, so much so that few could bear to be around him. What was needed was a firm hand by someone who could empathise with his problems and realise that this was not the real him. For survivors, it often seemed that a return to normality was only addressed once someone had bothered to listen.

The NHS seemed to be a collection of paradoxes. At times it provided some of the best care in the world. At other times, it seemed to me to sadly let down those it was built to serve. Similar to my private care, through my NHS journey, it seemed that the real challenge for a brain injury survivor was making sure that you saw the right person. As compared with private care, the issue with the NHS was that if there was a problem, it seemed far harder to change things for the better. Unhappily, with brain injury survivors, its ambition to treat those in need was slightly complicated as an extremely delicate touch was needed to deal with their often frail sense of self. There was the very real danger that if this was not handled with considerable delicacy following a traumatic brain injury, a person might lose their will to go on.

The death of ambition

Through my various medical appointments following the conclusion of my intensive rehabilitation experience, I understood that I had made an excellent recovery. Yet I still felt that something was missing, that I wasn't where I was supposed to be. I would often feel that my crash had not only dashed my head against the floor but also my dreams, as it seemed that all the stories of remarkable recoveries were reserved for others, not me. Playing with semantics and clever wordplay could only get me so far. Although in the past I might have had some smart, entertaining or sarcastic response to a question about life's troubles, this time it was different. In this instance, such an approach didn't work so well as the crash attacked the centre of my being, my ambition. As such, it wasn't something I could so easily shrug off. In previous scenarios, when I had been knocked low, my dogged determination would not let me stay down. In this situation I had been smashed flat and lost part of my face and would soon come to face a bitter truth. Even though I was surrounded by many people trying to help me, inside I felt so desperately alone and I lost hope for a better life.

Although at the start it was right and necessary for me to be assisted in almost everything I did, as I recovered, and as a return to normality loomed closer, I found that I would have to be prepared to fend for myself. As the training wheels came off, I came to realise that no one could be there to hold my hand for the rest of my life. My family would help as much as they could but it was still up to me to climb out of my hole and build my own stairway to heaven. My resolute (some would say stubborn) view was that that nothing was impossible if I tried hard enough – I could only hold myself back. Yet such optimism seemed grossly out of place in the reduced set of circumstances I found myself in.

As I flipped back and forth between hope and despair in the early days of recovery, I struggled against a damning erosion of will. At times it felt like I was not merely treading water and not moving anywhere, but instead I was actually being pulled back by the underflow. I was not getting any closer to the goals that I had set myself and the pot of gold at the end of the rainbow was actually moving further away. Such negative thoughts meant that I no longer viewed myself as the epitome of shining potential I thought I was during my premorbid days. My self-satisfied days were well and truly gone.

At times struggling against such pessimistic thoughts, it seemed that stretching out for my pre-crash self was by turns unrealistically hopeful, simply out of the question and frankly delusional. I almost felt that it was time to bury my ambition. Although my doctors were keen to stress that I had achieved an "excellent" recovery, this was by an objective standard, not the subjective one that I measured myself against. As the goalposts seemed to move whenever I glanced away, reforming my ambition just seemed so very pointless, not just some of the time but all the time. In such dark moments, I felt that maybe I should adjust my ambitions to simply being able to walk around unaided. I should forget about reaching for anything further. In an uneasy attempt to try and avoid such unhelpful thoughts, I would just stop dreaming about the future.

Although I had thankfully managed to escape The Bleakness, the successful resolution of this was not a magic bullet that would restore my ambitions to their pre-crash state. Even once I was out of the Wellington hospital and so avoiding the daily reminders of what had happened to me, I still felt something was missing. It was not something that I had left behind in the hospital but rather something that was littered around the location of my crash, like the various pieces of me that I had left behind in France. I did not want to just look like my previous self, but I wanted to recapture my missing drive. I didn't simply want to be Joe Blogs on the street; I wanted to be me.

As more time passed, I slowly came to piece back my shattered ambition. As part of this process, I thought I would just aim lower as there would be less chance for failure there. It was at this point that I encountered the double dip of recovery. Although I thought I had already dealt with the unhelpful and self-destructive thought that my life might never amount to much, I now experienced regression. Ironically, as I had done so seemingly well in my recovery and with a lack of immediately visible goals, I now had a bit of time to think. My idle mind betrayed me as it pondered circumstance and plunged me back into the nightmare of unfulfilled dreams. In such darker moments, with thoughts that I might never amount to very much rearing their ugly heads, I thought that maybe the best thing for me to do was to prepare myself for a rather incomplete, directionless life. I had come so far but perhaps this was as far as I would go.

As part of my attempt to bring some light to my darker days, I then thought that maybe I could learn a bit of perspective by listening to what the people around me said about brain injury. What a mistake. I found that preconceptions and lack of understanding could be devastatingly damaging. When people found out that I had had a bang to the head, reactions ranged from concern and curiosity to confoundment and pity. Yet regardless of their initial reaction, I found time and time again that the conclusion of their thoughts was that they would view me as if something was missing, as if I was less than a whole man. Although people tried to hide it to varying degrees of success, I could almost always see the question mark lurking just over their shoulders.

Such occasions would then encourage me to retreat inside my shell to lament the death of my ambition. I would ask myself again and again how I would ever aim for anything worthwhile when I was struggling so much. If life was so tough it seemed nonsensical to dream dreams as it could only lead to disappointment. It seemed prudent and self-protective to curl up into a ball. My ambition was reduced from the heady heights of being a smooth-talking lawyer to just being able to go to the toilet without assistance.

Although I had tried to address my lack of drive myself, it was so terribly difficult with the heavy burden of expectation. People expected me to be badly damaged now. They would not be surprised if I never amounted to very much. They would see my crash as an excuse to give up. In such a light, I felt that I had every justification to give up. It would be easier too.

Thankfully though, as the clock ticked ever onwards and I slowly regained use of my faculties and mobility, I found a bud of my ambition reforming. Yet it would take very tender care before it could blossom like it did before. The delicate flower of my ambition would need plenty of sunlight, loving care and most of all hope to grow. The first two would be relatively straightforward to work on, but the last would be more difficult.

When I had only really been exposed to people who were in the early days of recovery, it was difficult to see how I could aspire to create more hope. I had not seen examples of survivors who had managed to recapture joy after brain injury. I lacked examples of people who had managed to overcome the odds. So to address this absence, I thought it might be best to turn to books to see what others had said.

Other people's stories

As part of my goal to put bad things behind me, recapture hope and move on, I thought that it would be helpful to delve into what other people had written on the aftermath of surviving brain injury. I thought that broadening my perspective would help me put things in context. As an additional benefit, through this reading of other people's stories, maybe I would find inspiration or other nuggets of wisdom to help me return to my premorbid self more quickly.

Through reading other people's stories, a recurring theme I found was how others had dealt with hidden damage and how utterly normal they otherwise presented themselves to be. Through personal experience, I can vouch for this as once when I was out for a meal, a person I had just met was telling me about his friend's friend who he heard was in a severe cycling crash. He went on about how horrible it must have been and how he couldn't imagine the mangled person left behind. I then had the satisfaction of saying that actually, that was me. Many profuse apologies followed. This incident only served to highlight the general perception that there was nothing wrong with me that anyone could easily see. This was a blessing in a way, as people would treat me no differently from anyone else. Other people's lack of understanding provided additional motivation to continue to keep the damage hidden, so I should see it as forcing me to pretend to be normal. I became so good at this pretence that several years on from my adventure, I was a master actor at playing a normal human.

Through this subterfuge, I found that it was fascinating to see how people treated me after they heard that I have had a face-first run in with the road. I saw no need to advertise my life-changing event and as I read further into other people's accounts, I came to realise that reactions such as those I previously outlined were along the tamer side of the spectrum, hence encouraging me to keep my injury hidden. For others when they found out what had happened to me, they would recoil in shock and were left speechless. Others proceeded to treat me as a kid as if the injury had pushed my mental age back to five. Others treated me with a barge pole, almost as if they thought that my injury was contagious. The worst though would be those that treated me with pity. I could see in their faces that they were thinking, "That poor dear, doesn't he know that bicycles are dangerous, he shouldn't use those moving death traps." I had to fight the urge to tell them that walking around on the street is dangerous too. Tell that to people that are so interested in their phones that they walk into various objects. That's a good way to get a particularly embarrassing head injury.

The stories I read also encouraged me to try and help other survivors. As part of this I worked at Headway, the brain injury association, and through this I met numerous people suffering from the same "disability" as me. They all presented wildly differing levels of treatment and degrees of recovery. Some were like me in that you wouldn't be able to tell from brief contact with them that they had been injured. They presented as utterly normal. Others displayed very visible signs of damage, such as a walking stick or palsy, so it was easily apparent that there was something wrong. Unfortunately though, I found that, as was often the case with brain injury survivors, when the signs were more subtle there would be a lack of comprehension. It almost seemed that the only way that some glimmer of understanding in others might be achieved would be for survivors to walk around with large neon signs on their heads advertising their trauma.

So having decided to embark on my journey of self-discovery, I began canvassing the brain injury specialists I knew for suggestions of what to read. Through my prodding of others, I came away with a couple of suggestions. All were dramatically different from each other and came from people in many different walks of life. I found, maybe due to personal preferences, the British style of writing far more preferable to the American. In American writing, it seemed to me that feelings are worn on the sleeves, which seems to promote a more superficial exploration. Whereas, paradoxically, the stiff-upper-lip Brit is more willing to write about the turmoil beneath once they overcome the initial inhibition.

When reading these books, I found some were good, written by people who knew how to express themselves in complex but concise ways and those that were not so practised in this medium but wished to present an honest view. Robert McCrum, author of *My Year Off: Rediscovering Life After a Stroke* (2008), was an editor of Faber & Faber and later the *Observer*; he wrote with candour and wit, the way I would have expected him to before his incident. I later found out that he had published several books before his "brain attack," as he referred to his stroke, and so had some familiarity with the typed word. His example gave me hope as even after injury he continued to demonstrate rare skill in manipulating the written medium.

I thought to myself, maybe this was an object lesson that you could return to your pre-crash ability or close enough not to matter following an insult to the brain. In contrast to a literary critic such as McCrum, I also read other accounts from people in different walks of life. Their styles varied significantly and I thought this was a reminder that brain injury does not discriminate on the basis of education, occupation, health or age. A teenager cut down in her formative years in *Cracked: Recovering After Traumatic Brain Injury* (Calderwood, 2008); a magazine editor locked into his own body in *The Diving Bell and the Butterfly* (Bauby, 2008); a gregarious nurse who could not recognise her own husband in *Identity Unknown: How Acute Brain Disease Can Destroy Knowledge of Oneself and Others* (Wilson *et al.*, 2015); a professional athlete run over by a truck in *Touching Distance* Cracknell and Turner, 2013); and a conductor who could no longer follow the score in *Forever Today: A Memoir of Love and Amnesia* (Wearing, 2005). Each story was heartbreaking for a different reason. Yet thankfully all of the protagonists had managed to find some way to make the most of their changed circumstances. Through my reading of these stories, I gained a small measure of hope, as these stories were written proof that people who suffered an insult to the brain like me had actually managed to find acceptance and move on.

These stories helped me to understand that many of the issues that I had experienced were by no means unique. I was not some ogre who had been let loose on civilised society that should be kept away from children, lest I tried to stuff them down my throat when no one was watching. This is not as farfetched an idea as you may think. Apparently some head trauma survivors have tried to eat anything around them, rather like a small child, but with the important advantages of a bigger mouth and greater dexterity. This led to an increased chance of more problematic situations occurring. So a child may swallow a toy car, but what happens when an adult tries something larger and sharper?

The growth of my self-awareness through my reading of others' stories also slowly bolstered my esteem. When times were hard, it helped to be reminded that I wasn't alone. When things seemed too difficult, it helped to know that other people had overcome similar challenges. When things were impossible, it helped to see that maybe it was just a passing phase. These stories reminded me that I should not see the road as a never-ending journey, but rather as a series of short episodes.

Yet even after reading other people's stories of triumph, it was just that – other people's stories, not mine. Although my treatment so far had rectified some of my more easily treatable deficits, the construction of my purpose in my life was still very much a work in progress. By trying to fix my good eye on the manageable present and avoiding speculation on the distant future, I hoped to find myself at the end of the road before I knew it. As shown by these accounts, survivors were able to live fulfilling lives after an insult to the brain. I should try to see brain injury as a temporary setback. Life could still be full of many other opportunities for happiness and joy. I just needed a bit of help to see that it was up to no one but me to make it so.

The Oliver Zangwill Centre

Although it was the logical progression of my recovery to be discharged from the Wellington hospital, several months after my hospital graduation I found myself feeling a bit lost at times. Although I had benefited from some NHS treatment, this was an extremely limited affair. So, stuck in a no man's land between hospital and a full and complete reintroduction to the real world, I then proceeded to the next stage of my treatment, assessment for non-residential neurorehabilitation. The centre my family decided to apply to focused on traumatic brain injury survivors in a more advanced state of recovery. This was not to say that they concentrated on people who still remained "disabled" despite continued interventions, but rather that they wished to help people live a fulfilling life even years following brain injury and understand that life wasn't over after a knock to the head. Instead, it would just be a little different.

A place that had been lauded repeatedly when I had been in the Wellington hospital was a small regional centre in a corner of Cambridgeshire, in the city of Ely. In this city was a hospital that had a small specialist unit. Situated in this provincial hospital was one of the world's most fêted neurorehabilitation centres. The goal of this centre, named the Oliver Zangwill Centre, was to help patients reach their greatest potential, despite whatever odds were stacked against them. Actually, the use of the word patient is a misnomer. The people who attended the centre were called clients. For the privilege of attending this highly acclaimed "school," a substantial fee was required.

Due to the sums involved, after a referral to the centre, the NHS could be particularly difficult when asked to provide a client's necessary funding. Thankfully, it seemed that persistence sometimes paid off as the majority were funded by the public purse. Yet such a route could sometimes take a not inconsiderable amount of time. Thankfully, there was a shortcut to avoid this sometimes excruciating route, finding your own money. Accordingly, a number of clients were funded through compensation from medico-legal claims, whereas others with enough determination or other fortunate circumstances were able to fund themselves.

So this is why after striving for so long and with great difficulty to be heard by the NHS, I felt that my own convoluted path to the centre required some validation. I had to see whether there really was a pot of gold at the end of the rainbow. Fortunately, I was not to be disappointed. Much in the way that "Clothes make the man," the centre taught its clients that the best way for healing was for them to help themselves.

This centre accepted fifteen applicants a year and supporting these clients was anything from ten to fifteen therapists. The very high staff to client ratio was necessary for them to provide tailored treatment. Consisting of therapists from major disciplines, such as mental health, occupational disciplines, physical movement, speech and language and the clients themselves, the residents learnt not only how to survive after their brain injury but how to change the way they approached life. Their way of thinking was transformed so they no longer see themselves as disabled but instead throw off this label to become just like any other member of society. During my two-day assessment there, what struck me most when I spoke to the other clients was how cheerful they seemed. This was not a morbid sense of cheer, that things couldn't get any worse so why not be happy, but rather a genuine shift in their outlook on life.

This seemed to be a real-world application of the effect of modelling that I read about in Daniel Kahneman's *Thinking Fast and Slow* (2011). In this book it was explained that apparently unconscious actions can change your mental outlook. Holding a pencil between your lips sideways, thus forcing you to approximate a smiling effect, makes you see humorous things in an even funnier light. Described in Kahneman's book as the priming effect, apparently this unconscious influence on our cognition is undetectable by the individual in question. I tried this experiment myself but when I saw myself in the corner of my eye in a mirror in such a ridiculous pose, I promptly lost my pencil in laughter. As science explains, having a happy demeanour may increase your creativity and success in life. So modelling a happy life might lead to the real thing and eventually reality and the inner self might merge together to lead to a contented truth. In which case, it was time for me to start pretending then.

So eight months after my crash, while trying to find the centre, my family and I were a bit confused at first as, on arriving at the address provided, we encountered a stereotypical rural scene, single-storey buildings, a large car park and plenty of grass. This evoked thoughts of an idyllic countryside environment. We thought that surely this couldn't be where the centre was? However, we had trusted our GPS implicitly like all good modern-day citizens. The computer could never be wrong. We then noticed small signs scattered around the landscape pointing the way to the Oliver Zangwill Centre. At this point in time, I did think that maybe this scene was specifically designed to calm the nerves of slightly agitated patients.

The centre was named posthumously in honour of a noted neuropsychologist, Professor Oliver Zangwill, who continued to persevere even in this chronically underfunded and unchartered field of neurology. It seemed to me having been through the wars myself that specialist neurorehabilitation centres were too few and far between, especially those that provided care several years after the initial trauma. I guess that the issue here would be that brain injury survivors might not see what might be gained by further treatment only a few short years after insult. The tax man would also think that they would only be eligible after several years of trying. Why pay for something that might not be needed after all?

The Oliver Zangwill Centre was founded by Professor Barbara Wilson. Its goal was to address the mistaken belief that nothing could get better. It tried through gentle direction to put people's lives back on track. It guided people to viewing the world in a different way. During my time in Wellington hospital and through the literature I had read, I heard time and time again how the Oliver Zangwill Centre was the pinnacle of neurorehabilitation. So I had expected whitewashed walls, a sterile environment and expensive equipment in keeping with its eminent reputation. If the outside was different from what we had expected, it was inside where we were to find a greater surprise. We found a small series of rooms clustered around a central room with a worn carpet, mismatched chairs and a lovingly used and much-abused billiards table. Off to the corner was a lonely kettle in the well-used kitchen. Such an environment almost made me look around for the screaming crowd of undergraduates.

If the physical setting was so greatly at odds with my preconceptions, I was in for an even bigger surprise in regard to the social setting. The Oliver Zangwill Centre, or as the staff call it, OZ, only accepts candidates after an extensive assessment process to test whether potential clients would benefit most from their holistic approach to neurorehabilitation. Note the word holistic there, something we will come back to in more detail. Among other things, the assessment process concentrated on a client's potential to engage with the programme. An angry, violent or disruptive demeanour would not be tolerated. Neither would sullen silence. It sounded to me like they did not want to have to deal with a child in an adult's body. I got the feeling that they were looking for a willingness to engage and learn and compartmentalise emotions, looking for similar attributes that many selective schools target.

When the name OZ was explained to me as their short acronym for the Oliver Zangwill Centre, I had thoughts of Dorothy and Toto from

The Wonderful Wizard of Oz (reprinted 2015). I idly wondered whether, if I joined OZ, I would get a small dog too. Putting such idle musings aside, as I spent more time in the centre, I found this abbreviation to be rather apt. OZ taught you that all you had to do to come back to the "real" world was to close your eyes and metaphorically tap your heels together three times. What they were trying to instil in their clients was that many of the problems following a blow to the head were as a result of how you viewed the world. OZ taught you that many of the problems affecting traumatic brain injury survivors could be overcome through the considered thought of problems. Many of the issues that would cause difficulty or sadness were in the mind and so could be overcome just by thinking hard enough of ways to overcome them.

OZ gently pointed out that although people might perceive survivors as having some cognitive deficits, if survivors managed to mitigate these effectively and modify their self-image, they could get back to normality relatively quickly. A client's return to normality was not just a pie in the sky. Instead, if clients managed to change their way of thinking, their fairy tales could come true. They could go back to a normal life. OZ helped its clients address their problems in a compassionate way. It taught them to look forwards, to become better, rather than face backwards and become bitter, crying over spilt milk.

OZ strongly advocated holistic rehabilitation, which was the new buzzword in neurorehabilitation. It means that to deal with brain injury, one of the best ways is by addressing how it impacts all aspects of life, rather than trying to treat different issues in isolation. To my untrained eye, it seemed that the idea was that dealing with the client as a whole person rather than as a collection of individual problems helped clients to return more quickly to ordinary life; living in the real world did not allow for the artificial separation of activities. Although helping someone learn memory techniques was all well and good, if they were not able to apply it to their Christmas shopping it lacked probative value.

Alongside this holistic manner, I felt that one key underlying issue that the treatment at OZ tried to address was building up confidence. The idea being that once a client had built up enough faith in themselves, they would then be able to function as a "normal person" for an entire day. For me, disability fed to a large degree on my own insecurities and doubt. In hindsight, I have come to realise that a large degree of disability is cripplingly self-taught. Although a seemingly simple-sounding issue to address, I was to discover that it was a problem that only seemed to grow more complex the harder you looked, much like an intricate puzzle that looks so simple at first but grows to become breathtakingly elaborate.

Dealing with this perplexing mystery of confidence was of vital importance, as all other treatments could only really be acted upon effectively once this core element was addressed. As touched on briefly above, I thought that the high number of staff in the centre encompassing all major areas that might require treatment would provide a wealth of expertise to treat every facet of a problem that a client might have trouble with. Through this holistic approach, the aim was to rebuild a person and their psyche as a whole, a big picture approach to recreating a person and their image of self.

Once my family and I had been settled into the centre on my first day, my initial contact with the clientele was through observation of the morning community meeting between the current cohort of clients and their respective therapists. Here responsibilities for various housekeeping tasks were divvied out. From this study it was apparent that there was something different about the clients at OZ. Although my open surveillance of the clients was limited, I felt that there was something imperceptibly different about this group of people. At the end of my two days, I managed to discern what this was.

OZ had managed to recapture hope.

OZ encouraged the clients to move from wallowing in self-pity, to acceptance, to determination, to being content (I do not use the word happy, as that seems too strong a label) with their current state. Speaking to the clients when there was a break in the kitchen, out of sight of the therapists, these candid conversations were surprisingly revealing. There was no attempt to hide or brush aside difficulties they had had but instead what outshone their hardships was a determination to overcome them. Whether it was giving up a driving license, ambitious recreational pursuits or certain occupations, I was surprised at how acceptance had been made with difficulties. These people had managed to deal with their anger and sadness and instead move on.

To use a metaphor, I felt that my struggle was like seeing a cake on top of a high book case but promptly finding out that I was unable to assail said necessary elevation. It would seem as though I could not see any humanly possible way to reach the cake. Instead, the lesson taught by OZ was that I should stop frantically scrabbling away at the bottom and find some logical way to solve the problem. As I was told sometime in the past, the best way to deal with problems was to use the mnemonic, KISS. Keep it simple stupid. Best to use the ladder lying by the side in that case.

In connection with this message of hope, OZ also repeated the message that you should never give up. Just because you were unable to do something, it did not mean that it would always be impossible. Just keep trying. This unfailing determination to keep going was readily apparent as demonstrated by members of their current cohort. Although some had suffered from almost crippling problems, they were able to demonstrate that they could live a fairly normal life now. It drove home the point that if there was a failure, maybe it was just time to approach the obstacle in a different way. As the patience of the therapists showed, perseverance was sometimes more useful than IQ. It seemed that it was not necessarily how smart you are that is a reliable indicator of future performance, but how you pick yourself up after a fall. This was even more apparent as the clients at OZ had fallen so very hard.

Through this programme, it seemed to me that OZ taught a considered way to approach head trauma. What was particularly helpful was how many of the current clients were around my age, in the prime of their lives, and even after their own heartbreaking trauma, after some treatment at OZ they managed to regain their youthful optimism. Although at the stage at which I visited OZ, I was blind in the immortality of youth to this more reflective and mature lesson, OZ demonstrated that even amongst the anguish, agony and suffering of an insult to the brain, there is life beyond brain injury.

The idealism of youth

Youth seemed like a kind of excuse at times. He's young, he doesn't know better, he will learn. It also seemed to be some type of invulnerability shield as well. He can do anything. Nothing bad will happen to him. It will always happen to that other guy.

Although pointless optimism has its place, following my crash it seemed grossly unsuitable – I felt that maturity crept up on me with alacrity and I did not have the chance to wave goodbye to my carefree youth. Instead, it seemed that one day I went to sleep and the next day I woke up knowing that I had lost something. What made it even worse was that because of my limited self-awareness, I had only a superficial realisation that things had changed. Even this minimal awareness was enough for me at this point. If the full magnitude of how I had changed had been completely and prematurely unleashed, it might have been too much, too soon.

As time went by and I slowly came to terms with my injury, I thought that maybe it would be better if I didn't know what I was missing. The crash had crushed not only my face but also my dreams. To use an analogy, sometimes I felt it might be better if I was like a goldfish in its little tank. It can't remember that its world is so small because it cannot remember that it has passed this way before. Instead, life is a never-ending adventure because the fishy doesn't know better. Every minute it forgets everything that happened moments before. Just like me in my early days of recovery.

Once my memory improved, what stuck with me was the oft-repeated remark from others that I was a changed man. Yet I refused to accept such statements at face value as I was suspicious that they were making such claims for their own reasons. From within my own little world, I had no awareness of what things were like viewed from the outside. In such a context, the views of others seemed ludicrous and mad. In my artificial and restricted world I felt secure. In my blindness everything seemed fine as I was unaware of most of what I was missing. The piddling feeling that things were different now was ruthlessly crushed by me in the blindness of my youth. When others might hint that perhaps I was being slightly deluded and say that I was changed now and that I should just accept it, I would be driven into a temper. It seemed to me that they were saying that there was something fundamentally wrong with me. Anyone who dared to say I should be content with being a cripple would have to tread very carefully.

The more gentle hints that I was different would pale in comparison to the damage inflicted when people would say things could be worse, but as my awareness of the damage wrought grew, I could not understand how things could possibly be more poorly. My fury that others would pretend to know what it was like to be in my position would lead me to entertain thoughts of screaming. Why wouldn't they all just go away? How dare they pretend to feel what I felt? Empty words and meaningless platitudes only served to stoke my anger. The most cutting would be when people said that I was young and I would get over it. The attempted sage wisdom from older and younger people sawed like a dull blade. When people would say "I know how you feel" I would be tempted to use my hereto underused colourful language to respond. I felt that others were ill-placed to make comments about living with brain injury – they hadn't earned the right. Frankly put, if you hadn't suffered like me, go away.

Although I felt it was my right to rage against my lost youth, this self-pity was rather counterproductive. I slowly learnt that I could not let such dark thoughts overcome me if I wanted to heal. A more adult perspective on my situation would not mean that I would be kissing goodbye to my youth. Instead, I would be shifting my perspective to see this as an opportunity to grow in maturity and prepare for other stumbles in the future. As urged by many of the doctors, I should try to see the bright side of things. At least I was young, my physical healing was good and my mind was more receptive to different ways of living. The delivery of the message from doctors that youth has its benefits went down far better than from my peers and I slowly came to accept this message.

In this attempt to reframe things, I tried to see the post-crash world differently. With the benefit of perspective now bestowed on me by the crash, never again would it be boring to just sit and listen to the birds chirp. To listen to the water running. To feel the wind in my face. To taste and be appalled by badly cooked food. Life was so fragile and every moment was to be cherished as the blindness of my youth was stripped away. Instead I should just appreciate being alive and seize this second chance at life.

I should take advantage of the greater life experience brought about by the crash. Expensive clothes, fast cars, exotic holidays and other status symbols took on a rather questionable value as I bid goodbye to my rather carefree youth. Boisterous behaviour, trophy items and ravenous hunger for experiences would now be for younger people who had not been knocked down by life hard enough. Instead, with a different point of view brought on by growing up, I felt it was time to pause and smell the roses. And just be me.

The land of OZ

During my two-day assessment at OZ, what I found most calming was that I could let the facade drop. I wouldn't have to worry that I was being constantly judged by those around me. I found that the genuine warmth of the clients, the much-used but cared-for furniture and the lack of airs and graces by the staff created a sense of belonging. I could just "act" like me. It felt like I had returned home.

In such a sincere environment, I felt that I could revert back to my naturally inquisitive nature. Others might refer to it as poking the hornets' nest, but I preferred to call it an interest in broadening my horizons. When there was a break in the sessions, I spoke to some of the clients of the centre to try and get unofficial feedback on OZ. It seemed like the usual opener for clients at OZ was not "how are you?" but instead "how did it happen?" When I asked the clients, they would without any hesitation be glad to enlighten me as to why they were there. Causes of injuries ran the usual but no less tragic gauntlet of falls at work or in the home to the main culprit, motor vehicle mishaps. The age range of clients tended to be fairly young, mid-twenties to -thirties. There were no doubt incidents of traumatic brain injury affecting younger clients, but the usual cause, car crashes from driving at high speeds, required a certain level of income which youthful people might lack. I would also hazard a guess that the lower numbers of older people was due to age tempering foolhardiness with maturity. Further, in line with national statistics, the majority of clients were male. In fact, the group that was currently in session consisted of four men and one woman. I thought that the logic behind this might be that men tend to undertake more exciting, stimulating and risky (or foolhardy) activities more frequently than the fairer sex, so they run a higher chance of a smack to the head. I am reminded of school days gone by where my high school class would contemplate the best way to get down a hill. Without reservation, the boys would choose to go straight down and risk some bumps and grazes in the name of glory, whereas the girls opted for the more sensible (and skin-preserving) winding route.

Consistency was another key feature I was to experience at OZ. What struck me when I spoke to the clients was that they were remarkably steady and not prone to erratic emotions or behaviour. They did not swing from one extreme of emotion to another, although they had every right to. Instead they were rather calm and measured.

In particular, I noted that this peace with their situation could lead to more joyful situations. There was a propensity to joking displayed by one particularly verbose client. As the staff later conveyed to me, he was known to stir up the rest of his cohort, not just to cause trouble but to help by jolting the other clients out of their rather passive state. This also carried over into his interaction with the therapists. He was just the most obvious example of how the clients interacted; all of them displayed such positive behaviour in softer ways. To me this showed that there was no divide between the private and public lives of the clients and showed how they accepted what had happened to them and found peace. They were the same in all that they did. The same in that they were not hiding any particular deficits or weaknesses when in the public eye. The same in that they displayed a maturity of thought far beyond where I was at that time. The same in that they would not rail against the injustice of life, but were instead not hiding anything and just getting on with their lives.

Another clue to the different views of life after brain injury held by the staff at OZ was the particular methodology of my assessment. In comparison to the Wellington hospital, which concentrated on more standard analyses, I found that the focus at OZ was very much on functional assessment. Standard classroom testing was easier to administer and the results fairly straightforward to score. But what was more important to the staff at OZ was how I managed to cope in real life. For example, although isolated classroom examinations might show that my delayed recall was very poor, if I was able to collect the ingredients I needed for my meal by utilising external aids, then I demonstrated that I was able to compensate for my cognitive deficits. Likewise, if I was able to convince other people to do my work for me, functionally I might not display any deviance from the norm. There was no such thing as cheating in everyday life.

The more standardised intellectual analytical examinations would not be totally ignored as it was still important to establish an empirical baseline through exposure to a battery of neuropsychological assessments. The clues gleaned from these tests would then serve to supplement my Wellington hospital results. Alongside the functional assessment carried out by OZ, this more easily quantifiable examination would assist the staff in building an overarching and detailed model of clients to better formulate interventions. This more classroom-based testing ranged from the basic, "I'm going to show you these shapes, then cover them, then you tell me where they were," to the advanced, "Explain what this proverb means."

That is not to say that during my stay in the Wellington hospital, real-world applications were ignored. While at the Wellington hospital, one of the functional assessments was the purchase of certain items with a monetary and time limit. While participating in such a task I wondered idly if part of the examination was to see if I could think of a novel solution to the problem. In this previous assessment, I was told that the rules of the "game" were time limit: one hour; money: ten pounds; and outside assistance: zero. I promptly asked if that was all the rules, maybe I should steal from the shops then? That would overcome the budgetary restrictions. However, possible incarceration would affect the objectivity of the testing so I was strongly dissuaded from pursuing this line of innovative thinking. I was to act at all times in a normal and legal manner. I suspect that due to the relatively early stage that most of the Wellington hospital patients were at during their stay and the transient nature of their residence (with the majority being overseas nationals), it was just not suitable to treat and test them as they did in OZ. It was not as if the Wellington hospital ignored your ability to function in the real world, but OZ treated patients at a different stage of their recovery. As a treatment centre for people who were several years beyond their insult to the brain, the clients at OZ would have different problems to deal with. Subsequently, different testing and treatment would be possible and perhaps more valuable.

With the benefit of my previous examination results providing a bit of a steer, OZ was able to concentrate on my speech, an area of particular concern to me. During my various tests on speech and language before OZ, one interesting thing I found out about language was that apparently verbal comprehension is not, as a rule, affected by brain injury. If you knew 50,000 words pre-injury, you would still know the same amount post-injury. I had a lengthy debate with a SALT about the validity of this test as it seemed rather nonsensical that vocabulary would be an indication of intelligence when an individual's memory could be damaged, thus clearly affecting understanding. Yet after much discussion with the SALT, the conclusion was that in the absence of pre-crash test results, verbal comprehension was the most accurate although not perfect measure of premorbid intellectual capacity. Even if the results could be drastically affected by other neurological complications, the imperfect test was still better than none at all.

One part of my SALT testing at OZ that stuck in my mind was the twenty questions test. I found it practically memorable as it was extremely free form. More interactive than the probing I had received to date, I was instructed to ask the therapist questions to narrow down what word they were thinking of from a pre-prepared sheet which was placed in front of me. I asked again if I got extra points for creativity, to which the response was a flat look. I thought that maybe this was another part of the assessment, to test my recognition of non-verbal cues and this was to become something that they pointed out as being "sub-optimal." Before this exam began, I tried to ascertain the rules of the game. Could I ask the therapist any question I wanted? In which case, I asked what the answer was. Apparently there were limits, even at OZ.

While sitting these various examinations, I managed to observe in part the current cohort's treatment schedule. Through this observation, I got the feeling that there was something atypical going on as I noted that the clients did not have the slightly defeated look that I had seen in some other patients when I was receiving treatment in the Wellington hospital or in my local NHS hospital. When I managed to put a finger on it, I realised that it was because OZ had managed to subtly change their clients' outlook on life. One particular method through which I thought they might have achieved this was the use of semantics. Through this, OZ were using words to heal.

As an example, I noticed that at no point did they mention the "D" word. "Deficits." Referring to problems as "sub-optimal" rather than "deficits" at first did not seem to be such a great change, but on reflection I realised that they were so very careful to avoid any hint that things might never get better. Instead, referring to things as "sub-optimal" was seeing things in a gentler light. I thought that "sub-optimal" did not mean that the clients were missing something that could never be recovered. Instead, it implied that things could be improved. To me, this difference in semantics underscored how the treatment at OZ was so very different from other centres. Patients became clients. Deficits became sub-optimal. These subtle clues pointed towards the ultimate end goal that following a visit to OZ, brain injury survivors would become human.

Perfectionism

I have heard that the essence of being human is not to be perfect. Although I was cognisant of this truth before my crash, it did not stop me from trying to achieve perfection. During my treatment after the crash, I was told by my psychologist that trying to be perfect can be a very dangerous thing. When I first heard this I thought that it was garbage, as it has always been the motivation that drove me to pursue ever higher goals, a combination of carrot and stick. How else was I supposed to deal with problems if not strive to overcome them? However, as it was explained to me, it wasn't always good. Some type of limit needed to be set.

Against the background of brain injury, perfectionism needed to be seen in a new light. My life could not be lived the way it was before with an almost binary view of the world. As I was no longer blessed with boundless energy and enthusiasm, I would have to weigh up the costs of almost every single action. I needed to learn how to ration carefully what energy I had and build up my stamina. In time I might not need to worry about my reserves but for the foreseeable future perfectionism would be something to keep my good eye firmly fixed on. I would need to learn to accept degrees of completion as sometimes the pursuit of perfectionism could lead to things unravelling.

This was vividly demonstrated to me a bit over a year after my crash. I thought that as I had given myself what I thought was more than a sufficient amount of time to recover, I should be able to easily host a small dinner party with a couple of friends for an hour. Yet I found that the multiple interactions drove me out of the room in fifteen minutes. At this stage of recovery, I just couldn't cope with so much stimulation as it rapidly depleted my energy store and led to degradation in my mental function. I found that the most easily recognisable sign of this fatigue was my withdrawal from others. This was a slight problem when the party was in my house as I had nowhere to run. After this occasion, in an attempt to troubleshoot this slightly depressing event, I sat down by myself to review my performance.

What I decided was that in the future I would need to allocate resources where deemed most effective. I needed to scrupulously plan as much as I could. The unrealistic pursuit of perfection could lead to the derailment of the train that was me.

Through situations like this, I learnt that perfectionism deserves serious contemplation in a post-brain injury situation. At the start of my recovery, I found myself continuously doubting myself, worried that I had forgotten to check a certain point and then forgetting that I had gone through this issue before. It almost seemed like going round and round on the merry-go-round, getting dizzy and sick yet going nowhere. The pursuit of perfectionism did not seem to make sense for someone with compromised mental energy as to get the last bit completely right would take a disproportionate amount of time. In such light it was hard to see how it was worth it. From an objective perspective, the pursuit of perfectionism seemed to be a red herring, as fruitless as hunting for flying pigs. It was just a false promise of recovery as it wasn't a matter of willpower anymore. I could not through sheer stubbornness bull my way through problems; my body and mind just could not take it.

Even though I understood intellectually that I should practise some balance in my pursuit of perfectionism, putting reason into action was slightly more difficult. I could not simply snap my fingers and hope to change overnight. I had always been a bit more obsessive about my tasks than the average person. Friends would often remark, "It doesn't have to be perfect!" So to address such a deep-rooted aspect of my personality, some professional help would be needed to more quickly resolve it. Following a long discussion with my psychologist, I was advised to purposefully make one or two mistakes at first to see whether other people would pick up on them. They might not even think that it made a material difference. So as part of this experiment, I tried to change my habits in baby steps. Yet perfectionist traits were too ingrained in my psyche for a quick change. I couldn't stop being the way I had built myself from day one. A progressive change was on the cards instead. As I was to find out, my little experiment of intentional mistakes would help me begin to gauge whether it really was worth it to be perfect all the time. People might not even notice the difference.

Ironically as my condition improved, perfectionism became even more difficult to deal with. As a return to my pre-crash self became by degrees more and more realistic, I had to fight the urge to reconstitute some unhelpful beliefs, prime among which was the pursuit of perfection. Now, perfectionism can be useful in some circumstances but self-destructive in others. When I continued to discuss my single-minded pursuit of perfection with my psychologist, it was suggested that I find some other subject to devote myself to.

In this line of questioning, I explained to the psychologist that my whole trip which had led to my untimely crash was initiated somewhat by my need to escape the rat race of the office. I hadn't taken a prolonged break previously as I felt that I had to be perfect all the time. Extended holidays to me were regarded with distain. I had hoped that by undertaking something totally uncharacteristic, such as a long vacation, that I could return to work recharged. It did make me wonder though. Maybe getting to *almost* my pre-morbid self was just good enough. Although at an early stage of recovery I had despaired at reaching even a sliver of this, as my recovery continued to progress well, full reconstitution or near enough not to be noticeable seemed more and more attainable. I then questioned why shouldn't I strive to return to my perfectionist traits and view the world in black and white? It would make life a lot simpler.

In an ironic twist, I then found that my against-all-odds recovery was counterproductive. It encouraged me to return to my pre-crash thinking that what you did was either perfect, or it wasn't. There would be no degrees of completion, it was either done properly or not. In such an absolutist mind-set, I thought that perfect was the only way worth doing. As I was sitting down one day in the park, I found that things were actually not that bad. I could walk, talk and contemplate a Rubix cube. With some spare capacity in my mind to think, my inner voice then took the opportunity to steer me back to my pre-crash status quo. Unfortunately this led to depressing thoughts because when I contemplated things that did not play out as I had wished, I was reminded of things lost. It wasn't fair that things had turned out the way they did. I should be able to strive to be perfect again. In such a sullen state I would feel that my pre-crash life was simply a waste of time.

As the months went by, I slowly came to a compromise with perfectionism. I came to realise that not everything had to be perfect and instead I decided that I would employ my perfectionist traits strategically. It wouldn't matter that I hadn't ironed my shirt just right. Sarcastically I told myself that it was far more important to make sure that every *i* was dotted, and every *t* crossed. Things like being two minutes late for an appointment didn't really matter that much.

So with a better understanding of perfectionism, I resolved to apply relentless hard effort across key areas in my life only. I would tell myself that when I began to become a bit too wrapped up with a task, it was time to take a step back and reassess and judge whether some things were really worth it. The pursuit of perfectionism would not be so black and white anymore and life should be more balanced than that. Instead, I slowly realised that there were many other colours in between, a lesson which I could see that the clients at OZ had learned. Now it would be my turn.

The rainbow

During my assessment at OZ, I later found out that they had paid particular attention to the inner core of my being. Inside me, perfectionism, stubbornness and perseverance were vying with hopelessness, fear and apathy. To assess this inner state, the staff at OZ watched my every action, carefully weighting and measuring all that I did. During my brief two-day stint, the staff of OZ were hyper-vigilant to detect warning signs of a problematic internal struggle as it could manifest in a host of different symptoms. After my visit, on reflection, it seemed that almost every social interaction during my stay was carefully calculated to elicit certain possible responses to assist with painting their picture of me.

Although many of the tasks appeared at first to be testing language ability, the underpinning element everyone was keenly interested in was my executive function. To explain briefly, executive function comprises your higher level thought processes. Included within this area is an ability to inhibit yourself and stop doing things that might cause an issue, such as pulling your pants down in public. In a more proactive example, executive function is also the ability to plan activities such as assembling the ingredients and planning the steps to baking a cake.

Sadly, executive function deficits are very common among head trauma survivors and are fairly poorly understood as individual symptoms vary widely. As it was explained to me, executive function is thought to be concentrated in the frontal lobes of the brain. This part of the brain is particularly susceptible to damage caused by the whiplash effect of the brain moving violently forwards and backwards in the skull. The brain, floating in its protective and nourishing solution, is unable to adjust its momentum quickly enough when the head moves so violently. In such a situation, the inertia of the brain then makes it crash into the skull, which is unfortunately covered by bony ridges that can exacerbate damage. This violent acceleration/deceleration is typical of many head injuries, whether it be from the violence of a car crash or a connecting punch. So commonplace is this type of injury that it has earned its own moniker, "shaken baby syndrome," on account of the sometimes furious movement that would cause this type of injury. Young children being of a relatively compact size are more likely to be picked up and subject to vigorous movement by frustrated adults eliciting such damage.

It seems that there is hope though as the deeper science probes into the workings of the brain, the more optimistic possibilities are raised. One view suggests that executive function is not limited to the frontal lobe as originally thought. The circuitry of executive function is now thought to be distributed more widely throughout the brain. In my layman's opinion, this seems to make sense, as so complex a cognitive ability such as serious thinking would have difficulty existing in isolation. Instead, it makes sense to me that it would need to draw upon the entire network of the brain to effectively function. In any case, even though this particular theory is not accepted by all medical practitioners, I found that choosing to believe this view gave me hope. As explained by Norman Doidge in *The Brain That Changes Itself: Stories of Personal Triumph from the Frontiers of Brain Science* (2008), the conclusion he reached from his research into the brain suggests that other areas of this organ can compensate or take over abilities which were previously thought to be strictly demarcated. Apparently with enough determination and time, previously crippling injuries to the brain can be worked around. According to his studies, the plasticity of the brain means that it is able to reroute for lost function, overturning the established understanding that once you lose part of your brain, it is gone forever. Instead, the theory is that this dynamic and flexible network is able to recruit other areas of the brain to offset damage to one particular area.

This theory was all well and good but the true test would be whether this would apply to my situation. As part of this, the next stage of my assessment at OZ was for me to leave the sterile hospital environment, cope with the real world and interact with everyday society. I was asked to prepare a certain dish to eat, find out various pieces of information from the shops around town (without weirding out the various shopkeepers) and demonstrate good timekeeping by finishing all the tasks within three hours. I couldn't help but think that I was now the star of my own series of *The Amazing Race*. I managed to repress my impulse to check for hidden cameramen around every corner and shoved away a feeling that my every move was being watched and noted. This paranoia was not unfounded, as shown by the undercover stalking during my stay at the Wellington hospital detailed in "Standing on two feet."

The various errands around town transpired with a lack of incident. I admit that I was in a bit of a hurry as I was told to keep an eye on the clock. Unfortunately for the occupational therapist who was to follow me, there was a significant difference in our leg lengths, which made things efficient for me but not so comfortable for her. During my task and while tearing around town, I noticed that people would give me slightly puzzled looks. Not because they noticed I was having difficulty and wondered if perhaps I was one of "those" patients from the hospital, but rather because I was a man in a hurry.

Having completed my community tasks, I then returned to the hospital and transferred to a practical test of hand–eye coordination. This was a demonstration that I could cook something edible, so would not starve to death in the scary, food-scarce world outside. I noticed with a small degree of amusement that the therapist that had been following me around town seemed to breathe a silent sigh of relief as she passed me off to her colleague. She had to almost run to keep up with me during my excursion. Back in the hospital, her trial of trotting to keep up with me would be over. She could hand the "baby" over.

The next occupational therapist then introduced me to the kitchen. It was basic, functional and looked rather blast-proof just in case something went awry. Having finished unpacking my ingredients, I then began my food preparation task. Whilst cooking, I noticed that the new therapist kept on trying to engage me in conversation, which I suspected and later confirmed was an attempt to distract me from my task. Despite such diversions, I managed to prepare my dish without any significant upsets. Although I would say that I have a slight advantage here as my cooking skills have been forged in what I think of as a crucible. I did not learn at my mother's knee how to make *chop suey*, but instead I was self-taught in my university halls of residence, which had a particularly sensitive smoke alarm. The triggering of such a device would force the migration of over three hundred students out of their rooms into the outdoor assembly area, which would cause particular discomfort in the depths of winter. This issue would be compounded by a slight predicament, as you were supposed to evacuate immediately and not stop to fetch any warm clothing. In my university days, this did lead to some amusing episodes (for me, as I did not share the suffering) of fellow students wrapped in their towels, shivering and dripping having been caught in the midst of a shower. They would then be forced to stand on the sidewalk during a balmy day of five degrees. The responsible actor for setting off such a "drill" would then be given pointed glances and would have to watch out for revenge. Against such a backdrop, cooking a meal should have been as easy as pie. Well it would have been if the therapist would stop talking to me.

It was later explained to me that distractibility could prove to be a significant problem following an insult to the brain. Hence, the particular methodology of my testing featured constant attempts to try and disturb me while

I was completing various tasks; I felt at times like a donkey with a carrot being waved just out of reach. Such distracting actions did not have to be as great a disturbance as shouting at another person at the top of your lungs, but could be as simple as quietly (and seemingly innocently) asking for the time or discussing the weather. As I learnt through my neurological education, being able to consciously control one's attention underpinned, like fatigue, many other cognitive processes. The most helpful way it was explained to me was to imagine attention as a metaphoric spotlight. If the spotlight moved, things could be missed in the darkness. The lack of attention could hide many things, like the Lego piece stepped on with a bare foot.

Following the conclusion of my cooking task, I then moved on to a detailed exploration of mental health with a psychologist. I remember that in the past I used to scoff at the "head shrinkers" and think that mental illness was just solely what it was labelled, "all in the head." In my premorbid life I had trouble understanding how mental problems could so significantly affect people. I thought that maybe those that suffered this malady might just lack fortitude or perseverance. In my arrogance, I thought it could never be a problem for me. In the same way that I had discussed issues such as perfectionism with psychologists, I slowly gained a realisation of how important my emotional state was.

Although this view had already been challenged by my engagement with the psychologist at my local hospital, OZ did not just turn the tables but upset the flower vase, upend the chair and set them all on fire. My session with the OZ psychologist started with the usual social pleasantries such as "How are you?" It was soon to delve much deeper. When I was usually asked this phrase, inevitably it included follow-up questions about my health. When queried by numerous medical personnel about my general health and how I was, I was tempted to retort back when asked "How are you?" with a sarcastic remark such as "Sometimes I have to pay for friends so that's why I am talking to you," but I resisted this urge, as I think it would have caused some degree of consternation. "No, I am not well, why do you think I am here? You can go away now."

In this case, my automatic response of "I'm fine, and you?" was countered by the next question fired by the psychologist. After I had supplied the rote answer of "I'm good and you?" the psychologist quickly jumped in and asked me "But how are you *really*?" Cutting through the social pleasantries also reminded me of what my father, who is a physician, and a book by Henry Marsh, a professor of neurosurgery in his autobiography, *Do No Harm: Stories of Life, Death and Brain Surgery* (2014), have both said: that some patients would be caught in contradiction at the end of their treatment, being thankful to the doctor for being cured and yet having wanted to avoid being in the situation where they needed to be doctored in the first place. When they had finished their treatment, the more articulate and blunt patients might say, "Don't take this the wrong way but I hope I never see you again."

Following this more in-depth question, the psychologist then patiently dug deeper. Chipping away to find the underlying issues, she managed to unearth my major problem, my acceptance of the new me. With my old life competing with the new, mental real estate was rather scarce. As we explored this issue together, she explained that if I did not manage to come to an agreement with my new self, it would substantially affect the efficacy of all other treatments. What good would it be to have a perfect command of language but only be able to complain about how I was a sadly reduced me? An agile mind would be wasted flipping burgers. An excellent memory would be wasted on someone who locked themselves at home. At the end of this session I was mentally exhausted and I think my psychologist suffered from physical fatigue from the volume of notes that she had taken. So after this last part of my assessment, I was then left to my own devices for an hour while she went away to discuss my case with her team.

After a suitable interval, my family and I were invited for a debriefing on the assessment results. This was delivered by the neuropsychologist following her consultation with the OZ team. The report was the culmination of the various aspects of my sub-optimal functioning – drawing together the many different threads of my life. This tapestry was then used to extrapolate possible future problem areas. The rich painting also helped to provide a much-needed second opinion of my condition.

The report drew mostly foreseeable results but also some unexpected conclusions. Although I was objectively functioning very well for a person in my position, what I lacked was a "felt" element. As the staff explained, I was not able to fully grasp the consequences of my problems although I could spot them in others. In essence, I lacked self-perception. Although I had made some progress on this point, I still had much further to go. They were keen to stress though that this lack of perception could be addressed and would come with time. It was too early in my recovery journey for me to come to an amicable acceptance of my changed self. What they did stress was that my judgement was definitely not suspect. Although I could be by turns unrelentingly harsh or blind to why I was facing difficulties, my decisions were still carefully thought out and reasonable in the circumstances.

Apart from this very helpful debriefing, OZ did offer some immediate assistance. They would speak to my local NHS trust and explain in a hopefully more successful manner what treatment I would need. This seemed to be fruitful as several days after my trip to OZ, things just magically seemed to happen in my NHS case. OZ knew the ins and outs of dealing with the public health service to my great benefit. Their expert actions managed to open the door to necessary NHS treatment. Thankfully, my days of banging my head against a wall in frustration were temporarily over – something that I really didn't need more of. Suddenly things started to move.

I would be given the opportunity for neuropsychology, physiotherapy, neuro-otology, endocrinology, neurology, and speech and language therapy, all the treatments that I had been fighting for in vain before my visit to OZ. With these new chances to heal, I was determined to make the best of them. With the help of OZ, I had now managed to get past the seemingly rather obstructive gatekeeper and things were actually looking up.

An additional important benefit of my trip to see the wizard was that I now had two different sets of brain injury medical professionals independently arrive at the same recommendations – the idea being that while one opinion could be a fluke, if two people pointed the same way, it was time to pay attention. Although I had not participated in any substantive treatment at OZ, through the examination and engagement with the staff and clients, I grew significantly closer to arriving at the final stage of learning acceptance of my new self.

The last benefit of my visit to OZ was the relaxation of my family. The world did not seem as scary anymore as they now had a much clearer view of the journey ahead. The unknown path did not prove nearly as daunting when armed with such information. Although it would be a first time for us, we could take comfort in the fact that the road had been well trodden before and others had completed the journey successfully. We would not have to feel our way blindly through the forest and be pioneering trailbreakers but instead could follow the footsteps of those that had gone previously. So it seemed like at the conclusion of our visit to OZ, at the end of the rainbow we had found something more valuable than a pot of gold: the wisdom to go on.

The importance of semantics

During my visit to OZ, I took particular note of their use of words. They used language that implied that things would get better and were careful not to say anything which might imply something negative. That was of particular interest to me because while some of my friends have sneered at my use of clever words as my attempt to obfuscate meaning and impress others with my brilliance, my more modest reason for the use of challenging phraseology was simply that I loved words and they loved me back. Following my visit to OZ, I witnessed the real-world application of their use of semantics. To explain where my love affair with language began, it was with another little "adventure." When I was a little child zipping around my house I managed to do what most people say in jest – break a leg.

As a precocious eight-year-old, my resulting time in a cast was particularly torturous. With hindsight, it was a foreshadowing of my bigger "adventure" but as a young child I lacked perspective. At this tender young age temporarily losing the ability to zip around the garden while others were having fun seemed terribly unfair. Forced to sit still, at first I did what any bored and mobility-impaired boy would do, pester their parents.

Once this became particularly irritating, my father thought of a way to keep me from constantly bombarding him with questions. The particular avenue of approach he decided upon was a big long book with no pictures. Hopefully that would be difficult, time-consuming and give him some measure of peace. He thought it might also be good to choose a book with language that would stump a child. This book was *Lord of the Rings* (reprinted 2007) by J.R.R. Tolkien and thus my saga with words began. I initially found it oh so difficult to stop fidgeting as I slowly worked my way through the book with the help of a dictionary and an enforced command to sit still. Yet by the end I was clamouring for more.

This little hiccup made me a rather ferocious reader, so much so that I would often be chastised by my parents for hiding a book under my blankets. Books became a way to control and reward me. For example, for enduring distasteful activities like a trip to the hairdresser and being a good boy by sitting still while the barber snipped my hair, I would be richly rewarded. Not with a chocolate, a trip to McDonalds or a new shiny toy, but instead with the choice of a paperback from the nearby bookstore.

This love of words also proved part of the genesis of my ambition. Whereas other classmates would clamour for the sciences, sports or maths, I was happiest in English class. Other classmates would look on in puzzlement as to why I found such a seemingly boring subject so interesting but I found the rapier point and thrust of wordplay more exciting than physical success on the football field. For me, the story playing in my head painted through words was far more intriguing.

Encouraged by two particularly gifted English teachers in my high school, I soon discovered that I was not limited to reading other people's stories, I could write my own. My feeble attempts at visual arts could instead be compensated for by engagement in a medium that was better suited to me. Crafting a particularly meaningful sentence brought me much joy and allowed me to bask in self-admiration. I felt like such a clever little boy.

Through use of what I thought of was my rather extensive and varied vocabulary, I then started to develop a focus on semantics, which was only heightened by my subject of choice in university, law. Law has a particularly extreme focus on the meaning of words – so much so that a misplaced full stop might completely change the whole meaning of a sentence. An errant punctuation mark, never mind a misspelt word, could radically change the meaning of a phrase. As illustrated by Lynne Truss in *Eats, Shoots and Leaves* (2009), a mislaid comma could transform the meaning of a sentence. A different word could make all the difference in the world.

Working on this premise after my crash, I found that the same principle could be used as one of the ways to control my anger. This was as I felt that by changing words I could transform emotions. At first my fall from my bicycle was referred to by me as an "accident." This did not sit that well with me as it only served to fuel my rage; referring to it as an "accident" implied that no one was at fault, which seemed terribly unfair. Although I tried to dismiss such feelings of anger as rather unhelpful, I kept on coming back time and time again to the "accident." Simply put, I felt that I wasn't to blame. I couldn't accept that I was to suffer for eternity for something that I couldn't even remember. Even after I had seemingly put this issue to bed, innocuous situations would stir the embers of my rage and cause regression. A person happily cycling their bike would make me angry that I could no longer do that, then ashamed that I felt that way. A team in the park kicking a football would remind me of what I had lost and awake a longing. A child laughing gaily as they were chased by their mother twisted like a dagger in my heart. Other people's joy was poison to me.

After sitting at this stage for months, I slowly realised that the road to healing might partly be a way to let go and view things in a more rational way. I realised that it would be best to let go of the "accident" and move on. As part of this attempt, I thought it would be useful to change the way I referred to my life-changing event. I then resolved to refer to it as the "crash" instead.

I felt that "crash" would be a more neutral term and a more objective way of describing the event. This different word was also my attempt to decouple emotional elements. I thought that by making things more impersonal, I would be better able to control my rage. Yet I soon found out that life was not so simple. Although somewhat mistakenly I had thought that this would work, I found that using the word "crash" seemed too impersonal and counterproductively it breathed new life into the embers of my anger.

Ironically, "crash" seemed to mock the injury I had sustained by referring to it in a more dispassionate manner. I felt that the word itself was sitting in judgement of me. I thought that it was my right to be morose and sanguine about my face-first meeting with the road – life wasn't fair and I had every right to let everyone know that. Why should it be the "crash"? Why not instead the "unfortunate series of events"? If there was fairness in the world, why should things have played out this way? I had mistakenly thought that using the word "crash" would have the benefit of hammering home the message that it simply just wasn't my fault and help me move on. In my more rational moments, I had hoped that this change in perspective would be the final nail in the coffin of my anger so I could bury it deep in the earth. With this goal in mind, over time I continued to wrestle with this new word, but things were still not going the way I had hoped. I still was not able to let go of my emotions. As things were not going well, I thought that it might be helpful to try something else.

This next step would be to refer to the event as the "incident" – much in the same way that you would call a tornado an "incident." Although I refer previously to the word "crash" as potentially removing emotional elements, I later thought that it still seemed to imply that it was partly my fault as when people referred to their car crash, the implicit undertone was that they were somehow partly to blame. Maybe they had had one or two drinks so their reactions weren't that fast, or perhaps they were distracted by a passenger or had been busy texting on the phone. This would be despite the fact that the truck which actually ran them over was driving on the wrong side of the road anyway.

"Incident" was a slightly more effective way of referring to things than the "crash" as the word seemed to more successfully unpin me from emotional attachments. Neither did it hold any connotation or allusion that the event was required for growth through suffering or repayment for previous wrongs.

"Incident" to me didn't seem to be making an excuse for what had happened. It just acknowledged the past and did not attempt to make any assumptions about what had happened. Most importantly, it did not attempt to make any projections about the future, a particularly sensitive topic for me.

I found that I was stuck in the "incident" stage for the longest time. Although mostly devoid of emotion, it seemed to be a strained peace with the event. It wouldn't let me move on as it seemed to kick emotional baggage under the table. Several months on it dawned on me that attempting to divorce emotion from the most traumatic event in my life was not showing myself compassion. I was right to grieve. It was understandable that I was angry. It was expected that sometimes I just wanted to be left alone. The true injustice would be pretending that everything was alright.

As part of my internal debate, I came to a realisation that in order to move on, I would need to feel emotion. It was just that it would not be an uncontrolled outpouring of grief but rather something more controlled. It was just ignoring the problem to bundle it all up and leave it to lie forgotten in the cellar, never to see the light of day again. So instead I thought that a measured, careful response would be needed. As part of this progression I tried to reframe things from "incident" to "adventure." In this way, I tried to put a positive spin on things. Usual sarcastic nuances aside, I tried to reframe my perspective from it being a tragic, unlucky event to instead view it as a "character-building exercise."

Delving further into the word "adventure," I specifically chose it because it had so many connotations of positive elements. "Adventures" should be exhilarating, uplifting and journeys of self-discovery. Yet I would not delude myself that this "adventure" was all rainbows and butterflies. Otherwise the "adventure" would not be an "adventure." Neither did an "adventure" have to contain grandiose elements such as a monster to slay, a maiden to rescue and a broken crown to reforge. Sometimes the greatest among them all were those where the seemingly commonplace was made singularly extraordinary. It could be as simple as learning how to see again, making a solo trip to the corner shop and understanding when it was appropriate to cry. I thought that the greatest "adventures" were those demonstrating success amongst hardship, sadness and suffering. The most remarkable "adventures" could only be had by experiencing the contrast of life. If my "adventure" did not provide me with a different point of view, then it wouldn't actually be an "adventure" at all. An "adventure" would need elements impossible to overcome, inconceivable grief, the heavy burden of unattainable expectation and preposterous goals. Yet this would only make the eventual triumph even more thrilling.

So trying to reframe my experience of my own little "adventure," I tried to change my perspective so I would become the unbeatable hero in my own story. I tried to live my life this way yet against celebrations of handicaps overcome came inevitably crushing setbacks. As I dealt with problems and sometimes suffered reversals, I chose instead to view things in a different way. These challenges could instead provide a thread to my "adventure." Something to add colour and character. Something to glue things together. Something to drive home the point that I was an ordinary man with normal flaws and failings. I was not the invincible knight in stories; I was only human and someone people might more easily empathise with. Such failings would make my story more exciting as an undefeated hero was kind of boring.

As I pondered my unfortunate series of events, it slowly dawned on me that I had indeed experienced the "adventure" of a lifetime that had led to this unfortunate series of events. It was just in an almost unrecognisable way. Just because I hadn't planned for my "adventure," did not make it any less of an "adventure." Many "adventures" that I had read about did not start from careful planning, but were instead thrust upon the adventurer without their permission or any time for preparation. The most uplifting and captivating "adventures" were those where people overcame surprising and seemingly insurmountable problems. The abrupt and unforeseen nature of the challenge only made the story of eventual triumph so much sweeter. That was what made them "adventures" rather than fairy tales, as real life could be brutal, short and harsh. Fairy tales were also too unrealistic to empathise with and kind of boring for their lack of realism. A gritty story was so much more captivating, helped along with a couple of choice words of course.

Henceforth I was resolved to refer to the "accident," "crash" or "incident" as the "adventure" – the fantastic, unique and altogether rare experience of a lifetime. My chance to shine. My opportunity to make a difference. My privilege to start again. So I resolved that it would be the "adventure" from now on. That was the easy part. Now all I had to do was make it a tale worth telling.

The traumatic brain injury fraternity

Following my visit to OZ and armed with new-found hope, they recommended that I attend the local hospital's brain injury survivor group sessions to try and address my speech and language problems. The idea being that in such a gathering the patients could learn from each other. Although I was initially hesitant to participate, I later found that these group sessions provided much-needed perspective. They showed me that although I would find myself constantly railing against the impact of my short-lived flying adventure, things could have been much worse, as brain injury affects people in different devastating ways. I should count myself lucky that my speech and language issues were relatively minor, as would be shown by these group sessions. At least I did not display issues of failure of initiation, where some patients would display a rather studious disinterest in the world around them. Yet, this did not mean that the alternative, disinhibition was to be preferred, where some patients just wouldn't keep quiet. Other issues on display included tangential tendencies, going off on an unrelated topic, or circumlocution, talking around the subject. Sometimes, I felt that our group was like an ideal case study for speech and language therapists. Several sessions later I received confirmation that I had guessed right as we were soon assigned two university students who would gain valuable experience under fire by supervising our group sessions. This would be part of their course, experiencing the practical application of their subject. A couple of baby steps for them before being thrown into the real world, learning to feed the monkeys before dealing with the rather more ravenous lions.

My group consisted of a rather taciturn man, a more verbose male and a quiet and unassuming lady. Unlike the clients at OZ, the group was far more reticent to talk about what had brought them to seek treatment, although this may have been due to another issue, lack of self-confidence. The other extreme, wilful blindness, was also to feature. These sessions showed me how some people struggle with limited or no awareness of their problems. This was by no means limited to brain injury survivors. As we explored the issue of self-awareness, I thought that this was may be an explanation about why some people are so in love with the sound of their own voice. Maybe someone had tried to knock sense into them but it had backfired. Through these group sessions my self-perception was further developed.

I would be the first to admit that I am far from able to provide an objective assessment of myself as my self-image is constructed out of others' subjective perceptions of me. This was of particular relevance when speaking about subjective/objective perceptions of self. I thought that perhaps there can never be an objective perception of self as my self-image was doomed to always be an amalgamation of what others think of me. As my group showed, this was of particular importance in a post-injury situation.

Through these sessions, the treatment seemed to reinforce the underlying message of treatment that after a knock on the head, survivors should not give up pretending to be normal. As briefly touched on in "The Oliver Zangwill Centre," if I managed to model certain behaviour, how I acted might eventually coincide with the truth or close enough not to matter. This brings me back around to the issue of self-confidence, which is intrinsically linked with this point. Successfully working on self-confident behaviour in this way, I would then feel even more self-confident; it was a self-propagating cycle. Success breeds success. Similar to a snowball rolling down a hill, it gets bigger and bigger as long as it doesn't hit a rock or a small child.

Several weeks after visiting OZ, my NHS psychologist further discussed the importance of modelling with me in a more personalised manner than Daniel Kahneman in *Thinking Fast and Slow* (2011). She explained that if you are angry but modelling calm behaviour, eventually your actual state would reflect what you are projecting so you will calm down instead of giving someone the wrong end of the stick. So for me, modelling "normal" behaviour would be the best way back to normality.

In addition to self-confidence issues, the most visible sign that something was wrong in this group was that many suffered from word-finding difficulties. This was to prove my particular stumbling block too. To explain, let's say I was speaking to a person and wanted to ask if I could have a glass of water. I would have trouble finding the word "glass" and would instead get stuck. I might say, "you know that thing you put water in?" This is different from what people term as "tip of the tongue" problems, where they feel that they are almost able to grasp the word. For me, I would not even get that far. The fundamental nature of the word would elude me. It was of particular distress to me as I used to pride myself on my varied and wide vocabulary, as I further detail in "The importance of semantics." Indeed, people throughout the years had commented on this to my secret satisfaction. Having this element of myself diminished created a feeling that a massive hole had been opened in my psyche, so deep that I could not see the bottom. Who would employ a lawyer who had trouble asking for a glass of water? It would be like hiring an artist to paint your portrait but then discovering, after they had set up their palate, paints and brushes, that they were instead proceeding to eat and summarily digest all the artistic instruments and materials.

Having a way with words was so important to me that I pursued this goal with extreme single-mindedness. I tried many strategies to rectify this problem and although my group sessions were useful, they were unfortunately rather too artificial to move beyond the basics. Other strategies were also not that effective as reading words from the dictionary would put me to sleep. Doing crossword puzzles worked better for a time but I would soon give up as I lacked patience. Initialising discourse utilising a varied vocabulary was slightly problematic on occasion as a response would be required immediately. No one would wait a minute for me to find the word. Instead, I found that writing, as I detail further in my chapter "Writing," was ideal as there would be no time pressure. Therefore, I resolved to repair my syntax by reading and producing good prose.

I found this rather atypical self-help way of treatment to be by far the most effective way to rebuild my vocabulary and self-esteem. The rapier point and thrust of writing prose not only healed but inspired me. After many debates with myself over the months and as my experience of life after brain injury grew, I finally decided that I should write about myself. I thought that it would be such an interesting story. It would be fascinating to read about someone who had had a bang to the head. Another ancillary benefit would be that then people could stop asking me questions. If they really wanted to know about my journey, I could just hand them my book. I would not need to explain the background again and again to every person who didn't know about my adventure.

Writing a book about my experience would not only be part of my healing but would also shed light on what recovery from traumatic brain injury was like. The hope would be that it might help others in my position and their families. It would add a personal account of the aftermath of severe traumatic brain injury. Although this goal suffered from one small problem, at first it seemed like it might be too big a mouthful. Yet I thought that it would be the biggest shame if I accepted reduced circumstance as a get-out clause. So I refused to let it be an excuse. Just because it was difficult was not a good enough reason not to try. If anything, it was more of a reason to go on as few things worthwhile were easy and it would be such a pity to let my adventure go to waste.

So with this in mind, I decided that maybe I should aim for a different type of ambition instead of transient material riches. As shown by meeting other survivors, I was so blessed in my degree of recovery that I could even contemplate such a task. I had the chance that many did not have, the opportunity to give a voice to people like me. So instead of aiming for the stereotypical symbols of success like a fast car, imposing house and fearsome German shepherd, I should aim for a lasting legacy. A story worth reading. First though, I would need to put some bad things behind me, chief among which would be to confront the fear lurking at the back of mind concerning the Wellington hospital. It was time for a visit then.

A return to the institution

It took me quite a while to muster the courage to return to the Wellington hospital. The reason why it had taken so long was simple: I was scared. I felt a great sense of unease and trepidation when my thoughts touched, even briefly, on the hospital. I suffered from an almost supernatural fear but after a year of ignoring the elephant in the room, I thought that it was time to confront my personal bogeyman.

The journey of remembrance began once I stepped off the tube. The five-minute walk from the underground station to the hospital was very familiar, with the little shops along the high street seeming to welcome me back and the loose cobblestone on the sidewalk that had tripped me up repeatedly almost twitching in greeting. Lost in my own world, before I knew it, I had arrived at the hospital building. Fighting to overcome my general feeling of unease, I quickly entered before I could have second thoughts.

Once I stepped inside, I was immediately challenged by the burly reception staff. After letting them know that I was expected, I was then permitted to enter the premises. As my shoes clicked loudly on the laminate floor on my way through the waiting room, I glanced around and saw everything almost as if I had just left. As my gaze travelled the room, it seemed that almost every little object had a sad story to tell – from the well-used armchairs to the lonely looking rack of magazines extolling the latest fitness craze. I had always felt that those magazines were very out of place as they were in a hospital where people could not even stand. It seemed to be a cruel joke to display things that might forever be out of reach.

Teetering here on the edge of depression, I hurried further in before things could progress unpleasantly. It would be rather ironic if I ended my visit worse off than when I had arrived. As I took the lift further into the hospital, I entered the ward floors with shiny lights, slick floors and a liberal scattering of emergency buttons and cords. This was where I had spent my initial months full of despondency and it was pregnant with memories. I found myself remarking in silent surprise at many things. Had I really thought that the corridor was so long or the benches really so high? Was the hospital really that small? Wasn't the constant beeping noise really annoying?

When passing a patient on the corridor, I almost felt my courage desert me with reminders of unhappy days. I had to fight back tears as I was reminded that I was exactly like that before, a sad, blank and hopeless face propped up in a wheelchair in an empty corridor. As I passed by, I thought that facing this constant parade of broken humanity day in day out would be too much for me. I applaud the fortitude and courage of the hospital staff for being able to cope with this. I thought that willingly subjecting myself to working in such an environment would be too much. The sadness of the patients' psyches, with their sundered hopes and dashed dreams would quickly build to a tremendous crescendo that would be too much to bear. Although perhaps this was an object lesson that you can get used to almost anything as repeated exposure can dull the pain.

Turning to more positive thoughts regarding my own visit, I guessed that the staff would be curious to see how I was getting on. I thought and later confirmed that news from beyond the hospital was rare as few patients would ever return. This was not because they were scared of the Wellington hospital, but mainly because so few of them actually lived in London. Due to such diversity and the different origins of the majority of patients, as well as language issues, little contact was feasible. The therapists would then be left to wonder at what might have become of the patients, maybe inventing fictional stories of patients' future lives for their own amusement. This background was to explain the reception I was soon to receive.

Only one therapist had been forewarned of my visit, so for everyone else it was a genuine surprise that I had returned. Passing by a grunting therapist trying to manoeuvre a blocky piece of equipment, I suddenly heard all noise cease. As I turned around, surprise was not just written on her face but was almost bounding out. In her elation at the surprise reunion, the words seemed to tumble out of her mouth as she made a valiant effort to compress the months of my absence into five minutes of non-stop talking. The delight in her eyes was contrasted with my more restrained greetings. She asked how I was.

I replied, "I am good."

As we quickly swapped stories over things done and not done, I realised that I might have to try and get hold of others before they disappeared as it was approaching the end of normal visitor hours. I managed to unglue myself from her company by promising a repeat visit. I also passed her a box of chocolates so that she could have some tangible reminder that I was not a dream. I then moved further into the hospital to reconnect with others and to more fully dispel the unease of the Wellington hospital by meeting more of the staff before they went home. If that happened I would be left with only echoing, empty corridors, which might serve to remind me of bleak days past.

Although initially buoyed up by this happy surprise reunion, more melancholy thoughts were soon to reappear almost as if conjured up. It seemed that almost everywhere I looked there was something that would trigger some painful memory relapse that would erode my cheerfulness. Even as mundane a task as boarding the lift with its droning intercom voice announcing the floors reminded me of days of relying on just one eye. The many security doors announced to the world that the patients were not quite right in the head. The sleek floors hinted at foresight for unexpected accidents. The ramps spoke of design for those who could not stand.

As I moved further into the hospital in search of the woman who helped me to laugh again, I passed by a large machine with an evil-looking tube. I couldn't help but shudder in revulsion at memories of having this shoved down my throat. During this examination to see if I could be removed from my nasogastric tube, the doctors had to be confident that I wouldn't choke on normal food. It was up to the SALT to complete the envious necessary examination. The testing included having a camera stuck up my nose, down my gullet and having it wiggled around. I guess in some morbid way, it might be funny for observers but not the patient. I have the dubious honour of seeing up my nose, down my throat and inside my stomach.

I managed to eventually locate this therapist, who constantly seemed in a state of good cheer. Following her usual melodious greeting we then relived the more humorous episodes of my hospital stay. We laughed at cringeworthy activities she had had me try as she tried to get me to feel emotion again. Throughout our encounter I kept on thinking that she looked slimmer than before. When I remarked on this with appropriate decorum, she said that she had had a baby! In my mind I thought that that was particularly brave when her day-to-day job was filled with so much human suffering. I mentioned this to her and she was very amused and said her job was all worth it when patients recovered and came back to visit.

My final stop was to visit the man who helped to teach me about the new me, the neuropsychologist who had patiently explained to me how I might choose to mitigate some of the difficulties in my life. I found him in his usual establishment, a windowless office in the middle of the building. I guess that sometimes seniority comes with a bombproof shelter rather than a light-filled office. As we sat down to catch up over a cup of tea, he was eager to find out how I had been doing. As I explained that things had actually gone better than I expected, he was particularly pleased and said that he never doubted me. I waved goodbye with promises of regaling him with my progress in the future.

Yet there was one group of people I felt I couldn't miss visiting, the nursing staff. Thankfully, it was not too hard to find them. As I wandered up to the nurses' station, I spied a familiar head and as I approached this particular nurse's eyes passed over me with a glazed lack of recognition. I then waved at her slowly and a look of shock came over her face, which I childishly found rather gratifying. Following my identification, the various members of the flock were quickly alerted. Following the first nurse's cries of surprise, I then met the rest of my nursing team. The first nurse I met later explained that as I was so formally dressed, at first she thought I was a consultant. She had been initially confused as this was so at odds with my hospital persona. None of the hospital staff had seen me attired in more normal and spiffy wear as when I was in hospital, mobility was key. After settling the usual pleasantries, we then discussed news about the hospital, how the food service seemed to still be constantly on the precipice of disaster and before I knew it, shift change was upon us. I then made my farewells as it was an appropriate time to leave.

Having spoken to the people who had helped me in dark days, my feeling of gratitude to the Wellington hospital staff deepened and as I sat on the underground on my way home, I took an introspective gaze inwards. The return had stirred up many feelings and emotions in me. Throughout my visit it felt like everywhere I glanced there were reminders of how difficult the journey had been. If I had just been less fortunate, the cookie could have crumbled a very different way. It could have been me never being able to leave my bed, room or wheelchair. My life could have amounted to not very much of anything. I should feel blessed that I had recovered so well and my visit was the first step in the dispersal of the miasma I felt hung around the hospital. It helped immensely that I was only there for a visit, not for more treatment, and that it was not my home anymore. I found that that made all the difference.

Yet although this visit helped with much progression on my journey of acceptance, full acceptance still lingered frustratingly out of reach. As I thought about myriad different ways to progress, my return did prompt thoughts that maybe the best way to exorcise my demons was to write about them. As shown by the reaction of the staff at the Wellington hospital, I definitely had a tale worth telling. Writing would be the final step in putting such bad things behind me, demarking the line between past and future. Such a constructive pastime would not be so much starting a new chapter in my life, but showing that even with the shreds of my past life lying chaotically tangled in a mess, this just meant that I had all the threads I needed to weave a new story. I wouldn't have to scrabble around for weaving materials. I thought that writing something would be an excellent way to start my new life and it would also be my chance to show that if survivors never gave up, brain injury was not the end but just something new. So with this return to the institution behind me and this combination of my self-centred and noble goals, I resolved to put something down on paper. With my mind made up, now all I would have to do is write.

Writing

If there was one tool that I could call my favourite, it would be the pen. At times in my past, I held it with frantic energy in exams, with studious calm in boardroom meetings and with barely concealed rage when I wanted to stab it into people I thought had done me grievous wrong. After my adventure, I found another emotion attached to it. Putting pen to paper helped me to think and think calmly as words do not shift like other people's preconceptions, they do not have wild mood swings and they don't talk back. Most importantly, I wouldn't forget what I had written down. For someone used to dealing in absolutes, a fallible memory can cause *slight* difficulties.

Writing was also my way of ordering a very chaotic world when I was coming out of a minimal responsive state. A peaceful room with one person calmly relating their day sounded like the chaos of Shibuya crossing in Tokyo, the busiest crossing in the world with over ten thousand people crossing at one time. During my time in Tokyo, I would sometimes perch nearby and watch the people scurrying like ants to their various appointments. I would always note with amusement the hapless *gaijin* or foreigner who felt overwhelmed by this racket of traffic and people. They would stand lost in the middle of the chaos, frozen like a deer in headlights. In the early days of my recovery, I was the tourist in my own mind.

Small things such as the rustling of the wind could resound like the deafening bellow of a freight train. A simple instruction could sound like a cacophony of conflicting noise. In such a bedlam, it could easily become too much and the chaos would soon become overwhelming. So writing became my safe haven. My own little secret world I could retreat into when the going got too tough. A world which I could order the way I pleased and would not shift according to the whims of others. There would be no annoying dog barking in the background as I could ignore him and if he irritated me too much I could just write him out.

In this virtual environment I found that I could slowly challenge myself to grow better bit by bit. Writing was my means of escapism from my current situation. My perfect world where everything was exactly the way I wanted. There would be no inopportune interruptions, embarrassing events or otherwise uncomfortable silences. Instead with my world-building powers, I could reorder everything just the way I wanted.

In my own world, I could dream dreams again. It gave me hope as I could imagine whatever I wished and disregard my diminished circumstances. Although I might only be able to advance in staggering steps from my chair to my bed, in my writing I could break the four-minute mile. My writing was where I could confront everything on a level playing field. If I wanted to be superman, all I had to do was write it. If I wanted to change history, I could do it with the stroke of a pen. If I didn't like things, I could just cross them out.

Writing also fulfilled a practical element as it helped me to overcome my speech impediment, the word-finding problems further detailed in "The importance of semantics" and "The traumatic brain injury fraternity." In writing, unlike the real world, I could sit and meticulously select my words. A response with an eloquent reply need only be made when I was ready. I could spend as much time as I wanted to find the perfect word. Writing took the edge off pressure as it was much easier to enunciate myself without the added complication of stage fright. I particularly hated being stumped for words, which was only exasperated by stress. Standing there grasping for words, I looked like a fish out of water as I futilely searched for the right word to fill the silence. Fortunately for me, my practice in a written medium soon transferred into verbal delivery. I grew into what I thought was a hallmark of an educated and eloquent person, being able to provide a spontaneous witty reply.

So writing provided many benefits. It helped me with ordering my life, rebuilding my dreams and being more articulate in person than on paper; the world was the way I wanted. Through my writing I could be anyone I wanted to be. As an additional benefit, I thought that in my rewriting of myself that maybe if I was lucky, who I wrote and who I was now might merge together and become the truth. This writing would also be my chance to show the world after brain injury, that life could still be full and fulfilling. Now that was truly something worth writing about.

Excuses and choices

Attempting to view the world in a more upbeat manner, I tried to change my perception of my adventure to opening up hitherto new vistas and horizons for my life. Such a view seemed to become increasingly justified as my recovery went from strength to strength. As my recovery continued to progress excellently, I now had the chance to make of my life what I wished. I would now have the opportunity to decide how my future would play out.

So my new life presented two choices. Either I could go back to my pre-adventure self and pretend nothing had happened, or I could make the most of this chance to start anew. Whereas in the early days of my recovery, I was very much focused on trying to regain a modicum of normality, now that I was almost there, my priorities changed. I had a choice, I had a chance to take a breath and decide what I wanted to be. Would I continue to reach for the stars? Or instead be content and simply watch others fulfil my dreams?

One key issue I found myself musing over for the longest time was my future working career. I felt that if I returned fully to my pre-adventure job that would be recognition that my adventure had not negatively affected my intellectual capacity. Yet a return to work was fraught with numerous potential pitfalls. The danger was that if I attempted to return to work and failed I might be seen as having a critical deficiency, face ridicule or worse still be constantly reminded of what I had lost. There was a possibility that trying but being defeated might crush my spirit. A safer alternative could be stepping away from being a lawyer, even though that was all I had ever known. Thankfully supported by my bosses at work, I was fortunate that they were prepared to explore other alternatives. They raised the possibility of changing to a less stressful position. Yet such a change would mean stepping away from something I had spent my entire working life being, saying goodbye to the high-octane and intellectually demanding profession of being a solicitor.

Although this safety net was very much appreciated, I rejected such a get-out immediately with much violence. I could not stomach such a massive change in circumstance and I refused to make a conscious decision to run away from a challenge. It was repugnant to live what I saw as an unfulfilling, aimless and most of all wasted life. It would be abhorrent and a disservice to my against all odds recovery, the tireless work of the various medical professionals and the suffering of my family, a squandering of the opportunity that I had been given. It would be the height of bad taste to glaze over my adventure. Unlike many things that had happened to me on my adventure, here I had the freedom to choose.

So I resolved to pursue a return to work with singled-minded devotion. As part of this preparation I would squirrel myself away with exercises and pretend work; yet this was not enough, as my interactive skills with others could not be simulated. This particular worry, combined with fears shared by my doctors that due to the nature of brain injury, there were limits to what they could predict might go wrong next, meant my return to work would be stepping into the great unknown. Although I was buoyed up by the apparent ease and familiarity of the exercises I managed to complete, the nattering in my head continued. It was almost the same conundrum that I had faced in hospital as simulation was just that, not real. So the voice in my head tried to scare me that it might be me shattered on the floor in a million pieces if I embarked on this course of action. Too soon and too fast might be enough to break me.

On my good days such worries would seem to fade into the background. On my bad days they bludgeoned me with thoughts of being a failure. On the worst days they made me want to curl up in a ball and hide in a closet. They breathed almost inaudibly in my ear that as remarkable and atypical as my recovery had been, this might be a step too far. I might not make it. It might be most sensible to give up now.

In this whirlwind of feelings, another emotion came to the fore and subdued the storm, pride. In the same way that it had propelled me out of my wheelchair and to my feet, it whispered to me that I wouldn't be able to stomach a life empty of meaning. The murmur continued to slowly wear away at the niggling fear at the back of my mind. The prideful voice murmured that I couldn't walk away if I hadn't even tried. If I did not make an attempt, the rest of my life might be full of what ifs and maybes. A more cursed existence was hard to imagine. Now that would be true defeat, giving up when I hadn't even begun.

Excuses and choices. I had been handed an almost *carte blanche* by my adventure. No one would have justification to blame me if I gave up. In my return to work, I would undoubtedly struggle against seemingly insurmountable hurdles, attempting to overcome prejudice and preconceptions of brain injury. At times it seemed like everyone was an expert at brain injury, they would lecture with authority on what an insult to the brain entailed even if their knowledge was from Hollywood. Yet, I chose instead to see things in a different light.

I made the choice to see my return to work as an unimaginable advantage, as I would almost have a premonition of what was to come. I would almost have the benefit of a crystal ball in my journey to return to work as it would not be like starting work again for the first time but working with a foresight of what lay ahead. So with such an edge, I then began to feel that it would be criminal not to make the attempt. With such a singular advantage, my choice was clear. It would be unthinkable not to try again. So against such a backdrop, I could do nothing less than dust off my jacket, tie my shoes and step out the door.

A constructive pastime

If you had asked me just before my adventure what I thought about work, I would have said I needed a bit of a break. As my adventure was soon to show me, I would definitely get that and more. Through my character-building experience, with its many ups and downs, I learnt to view life from a different perspective. So with this tilted point of view, I found that work became a pivotal point in my new concept of self. I longed for it as I saw it as my ability to give back to a world that had helped me recover and as an unspoken challenge to prove that the suffering, fear and uncertainty about my future was just unsubstantiated worry. Work would be my opportunity to show the world that after brain injury, survivors could still be constructive members of society.

I remembered how as a little boy on Christmas Eve I would sit with almost unbridled anticipation awaiting presents from Santa. My desire to return to work was scarcely less. In preparation for my return, I wiped down my briefcase, aired my suit and ironed my shirts. I took out my shoes and polished them to a never before achieved shine. I made sure to pack my handkerchief so I would be poised for anything that might come my way. Although this might seem slightly too enthusiastic for a return to work, I felt that it was such a major event as in the months following my adventure I had been given such a tiny chance of ever daring to step back in the door. It would be my chance to show that I had overcome my adventure.

Although I yearned to return to the office and had prepared all external elements so methodically, I also dreaded it and ironically preparation only served to exacerbate the worry. As the first day of the rest of my life approached, I began to have misgivings about my return as the corporate world is famously unforgiving and harsh. I worried that if I was thrust straight back into the thick of things and was unable to perform, I would be thought of as lazy, stupid or a combination of both. I was also very concerned about how people would react to my reappearance. Would the stigma of "brain injury" haunt me wherever I went? Would I be viewed with pity? Would people think I was a lesser man?

I need not have worried so much. Leaving home on my first day with my bags packed, my tie done just so, I soon arrived at the imposing stone and glass office. On this day with an empty briefcase instead of a full lunch box, as I walked in the office doors there was nary a whisper. No one was there to greet me. Rather I joined the crowd of suits hurrying to their desks. Although it was so symbolic an event to me, it felt like the world trundled on unperturbed and uncaring.

When I arrived back on my office floor and met colleagues in the corridor, at their desks or near the proverbial water cooler, most seem to studiously ignore my time off. They asked me how my weekend was, as if I had only been away for a couple of days, not the absence of more than a year. At first, I thought that it was a lack of interest and that no one cared. Later, I came to realise that my colleagues were actually doing me a great service. They were pretending nothing had happened, so in their kind way suppressing their curiosity and refusing to dredge up bad memories. This behaviour of ignoring the elephant in the room also had another benefit: it encouraged me to practise being normal.

So following the first day's excitement, I went home elated. It did not matter that I had not managed to do anything particularly constructive. That would come in due course and it was sensible not to hurry things. Instead, I took heart in that I had managed to reach further than my wildest dreams. In the same way that many of my triumphs of recovery had come, banishing the wheelchair, saying goodbye to the hospital and attaining full awareness, the day of my greatest victory came upon me with a lack of spectacle.

Prior to my reappearance at the office, a significant amount of preparation had been done. There had been almost endless discussions between my doctors and my employers. The very real concern was that if this was not handled with appropriate delicacy, things could go south quite fast. My recovery had been mapped out with particularly judicious planning and I was extremely fortunate that my work was willing to go far beyond what was strictly necessary for an injured employee.

Following on from my first day, my work progressed from a slow three-hour day, three times a week, before building incrementally to a normal nine-to-five job and then full unrestricted hours. My employers were keen to take the doctors' advice on board and kept in mind the warning that my return could potentially take months and possibly even years. Neither should any particular stumbles be seen as critical failings that might never be resolved. Instead, it was stressed that as brain recovery can continue indefinitely and sub-optimal actions compensated for, the most important thing was to help the survivor keep a positive frame of mind.

As time went by and my hours were slowly built-up, I owe immeasurable thanks for the aplomb, support and patience displayed by my colleagues and in particular two bosses during these challenging times. Together they ensured that through a steady and measured process, I was able to return to full-time normal work. In the early days of my return, they treated me with particular deftness to avoid me failing and falling on my face. That would be less than ideal given my history. In latter days when the training wheels came off, they ensured I could trundle down the road happily and safely on my own, avoiding any potholes or errant vehicles.

Yet through my discussions with other survivors, I realised that I had had a particularly supportive work place and an atypically quick recovery. I had heard many stories of how things could go horribly wrong. If things were not handled with particular caution, a return to work could end up like a car crash. It seemed that many employers had a short-term view, lacked patience and were ready to write off employees rather quickly for any perceived failings. This mistaken belief seemed to be that brain injury survivors were more work than they were worth. However, given my experience, I thought that that was a sadly mistaken view. If given the chance, survivors would be so keen to return to a constructive pastime that they would contribute in unexpected and helpful ways, have an alternative point of view and might be hardier than other employees and more willing to push on in the face of difficulty. Most importantly, as something which seemed to be rarer in today's transient job economy, if handled correctly an employer might gain something money could not buy, a dedicated, committed and enthusiastic employee.

I was so caught up in my recovery that once I restarted work, time passed rather quicker than I expected. So this was how almost a year after my reintroduction to work and after I had been on full hours for several months, I paused a moment and contemplated how my life had played out. Now that I was back doing normal work, I found that it was the last piece of the puzzle of returning me to me. Through work I found I could function again as a valued member of society and earn my bread like any other normal person. In the work place, I found that worries gnawing on my mind and concern that my new fragile concept of self might be swept away were unfounded. Instead, I felt that my self was stronger even for just trying.

Although at first I had to concentrate hard to act normal, especially with others watching intently, after a while things became easier. Time proved to be the great healer and as the clock ticked onwards, it seemed that people forgot my adventure. So this was how after a while I did not have to feign indifference to my situation anymore. I didn't have to pretend to be normal. I actually was.

When this realisation dawned on me, it did cross my mind to make some type of theatrical celebration but I thought that would be slightly too melodramatic. I thought that a private celebration and more subdued jubilee might be more in order. So this was how at three p.m. I found myself in the office canteen sitting in front of a slice of cake. In this less than dramatic environment, with empty tables, TVs quietly murmuring the financial news in the background and forlorn empty tray racks, I had some cake. Although it almost seemed like a replay of my birthday in hospital, there was a fundamental difference this time. Instead of tasting like opportunities lost, the cake now whispered of chances to come. I had now accepted that I was a changed man, not less, not worse, but with different but no less ambitious dreams. I found that I had now arrived at what I had thought throughout my recovery was a tantalisingly frustratingly out of reach goal, full acceptance. Now that deserved another bite.

An unexpected but welcome opportunity then arose to test how much I had recovered by secondment to another work place. Here was a chance to make a splash in a pond where no one would know my history or compensate in any way as they couldn't know; it would also be another challenge to overcome. Although I was initially apprehensive about this new work environment, once I was in it, I found that I actually rather enjoyed it as I could act just as myself and just be another lawyer. Guided by two particularly helpful bosses during this opportunity, I found that rising to the challenge and succeeding was the sweetest victory there was. I couldn't have thought of a better test and at the conclusion of this secondment and at my debriefing, in typical British fashion, nothing much was said. Things were going swimmingly then.

Following this, I then returned to private practice and joined the ranks like any other employee. Life was looking up. So this was how almost two years after I started back at work, I met with my occupational physician for what was to be my final check-up. We had kept in constant contact during my return to work with periodic meetings to keep abreast of the latest developments. As such, he was intimately aware of my career, especially given his experience in returning finance professionals to work following serious head injuries. At this appointment, we found that atypically we were running out of things to say.

At previous meetings, we would be so deep in conversation that we would need a bit of a prod to finish up in time for his next patient but things today seemed a bit more quick and straightforward. From the various reports he had received, it was clear that I could now cope with a time-pressured environment, frantic tasks and agitated clients. Most importantly, no one had raised any issue with my work as I was being treated just as anyone else would be with normal demands and pressures. It seemed like I was pretty good at being normal then.

At this stage, he mentioned his very pleasant surprise at the extent of my recovery. When he had read my medical reports before he first met me to discuss a return to work, he admitted that he had little cause for optimism given the seriousness of the trauma. Yet, as I was later to discuss with other doctors, my secret ingredient for success was simple, the determination to go on.

Through my character-building exercise I had come to realise that although reality might not readily submit to my will, what I could change with expeditious speed was how I perceived things. If I found things difficult, I tried to see it as a challenge. If I failed at something, I tried to view it as an opportunity to think of an alternative approach. If I had learnt anything from my adventure, it was that the most important thing in life was a determination to never give up. So if things did not turn out the way I had wished, I would try, try and if I had more time, try again.

With the end of our meeting approaching, my doctor and I discussed new beginnings, and how it seemed that I was coping more than well with things. His medical opinion was that he could see nothing further to be gained from additional appointments. It would now be an appropriate time to consider discharge. That would give a message to the world that all was well as he could see no reason for me to be treated differently from anyone else now. Although I remarked that I would miss our interesting chats, it would be time for me to discard my last crutch, him.

As I prepared to leave our last appointment, I packed up my bag, slotting everything away in its correct spot, pen here, notebook there, much as if I was filing away memories. When I zipped up my bag with its neatly sorted contents, it felt like I was firmly closing the book on this chapter of my life. I paused as I opened the door to leave as I was sorely tempted to say "I hope you don't take this the wrong way but I hope to never see you again" but I held my tongue. If my experience has shown me anything, you never know what the future might hold. So instead, I shook his hand, thanked him profusely and walked out into a sunny, warm day.

An (almost) new start

There is definitely a much more fulfilling life to be had than chasing dreams. Living them.

Here I was almost at the top of Thorong-La Pass in Nepal. As I climbed the steps to a higher elevation, I could only think of things to come. As I took my final ascending step, I realised I was finally in Thorong-La Pass, the highest mountain pass in the world at 5400 metres. The day had started at a balmy negative fifteen degrees and progressed to have the sun mercilessly beating down after a four a.m. ascent. It was the whole reason for this little adventure to Nepal, the culmination of a father–son trip, reaching even higher than Everest base camp. Arriving at the top was testament to the success of both of our preparation for physical torment when the pain became bad and our mental fortitude when we were tempted to give up.

Our training paid off as my father was among one of the first trekkers to make it to the top, passing numerous younger hikers along the way, proof that even in physical feats, sometimes old wisdom and tenacity can trump youthful exuberance. The sometimes torturous, often gruelling, but always exciting trip through the mountains on the way to the pass was a great builder of perspective. By day we would endure the steady up and down as we climbed ever closer to our end goal. By night we would lapse into exhausted sleep, huddled in our sleeping bags against the bitter cold. We found that normal life was even sweeter with such contrast.

As we treasured our accomplishment from the top, I thought that the view of Buddhist prayer pennants fluttering in the sometimes blustering gale and gentle breeze was an apt reflection of the extremes of life. We would never forget our time on top of the world as the experience was seared into our brains by the lack of oxygen at these heady heights. Above many clouds, the bleak, destitute and barren landscape seemed even more beautiful as this alien, dead pass served to remind us of the pain needed to reach it. This was a journey worth writing about.

Yet the adventure would not stop there as after this we would look forward to seeing the elephants, rhinos and tigers while on safari in Chitwan, and then I would be dropping by Doha on the way home to London for a bit of retail therapy. So much to look forward to! Yet the most important thing was that this time, it was not a dream.

This is what really happened.

I wish I could end with a pithy one-liner but that would be doing my adventure a disservice; it could not be so easily compressed like that. Now, with such a breadth of experience to frame things, life could be more objectively assessed. My adventure had granted me the privilege of starting again from a blank slate and with the benefit of hindsight. I now had the chance to reshape myself into anything I wanted to be. My adventure was my license to be different.

So with my old life ended and a new opportunity there for the taking, I was determined to make the most of my adventure. It would be up to me how I would view my past and what I would make of it. As thoughtfully put by Harold Kushner in *When Bad Things Happen to Good People* (2002), this was my chance to make an infinitesimal change in the world by maybe helping people understand. I could try and lead by example, showing the world that brain injury did not mean hope died. I would strive to be better rather than bitter. Instead, a hard knock on the head should be seen as a new beginning, the start of a new adventure, rather than the death of everything known.

My adventure reframed my life as I got a longer break than I wanted in an exciting, thrilling and unexpected manner. Through this I would gain perspective in a rather abrupt way. I learnt what it was like to lose hope, hit rock bottom and have my very soul undermined. I experienced what it would be like to relive my formative years at high speed with sadness-tinged joy. I learnt what was really important.

With such "exciting" experiences, once I was back at work, I gained a different view about my occupation. I approached each day in my office with joyful anticipation of problems to come and viewed challenges as hurdles to vault. Initially I thought that my enthusiasm would maybe be fleeting and would fade after the novelty of being useful wore off. Yet the sense of value and purpose continued to persevere as I saw things with the benefit of a different point of view.

When people ask me what I learnt from my adventure, I reply that it is the value of an alternative point of view, gaining a different perspective of life after brain injury. I came to understand that I should treasure what I had now and not yearn for a speculative future. I learnt that living a mundane, ordinary life could be a thrilling adventure. I now rejoice in being able to simply stand on my own two feet, taste bad food and deal with agitated clients.

Although I have had to bid farewell to my more adventurous hobbies, to my great sadness, I comfort myself with the knowledge that I am still able to enjoy more important things in life.

My adventure also provided another benefit; it helped me grow up far more rapidly than I would have otherwise. Now I feel wise beyond my years with this new maturity and new-found understanding of what is most meaningful in life. It almost feels that when I wake up each day, I have been blessed with an unusual degree of clarity. This new perspective sometimes makes me feel like an old geezer in a young man's body. The old man inside had lived so many "interesting" experiences as he grew up again, hopefully not to be repeated. The young chap would see the world in a more realistic light with a catastrophic incident that put everything in context. Through the forceful union of the old geezer and the young lad, the new me was able to view the small annoyances and sometimes larger problems of life in a more realistic light. Life was what you make of it and I choose to make it better.

Through my adventure I also fulfilled one of my life's ambitions in a roundabout way – writing a story. This more self-centred goal would be balanced by a desire to bring some measure of understanding and comfort to others who have or are suffering through desperate days following a traumatic brain injury. I also hope that it provides some small degree of understanding for those who come into contact with survivors of a blow to the head. Although I am not so arrogant to think that my story might lead to a eureka moment of understanding; instead, I would be more than content with even a small change such as a more gentle, compassionate, and empathic appreciation of the effect of an insult to the brain. Perhaps others will hear a whisper of what living with smashed goals, an unwillingly wrenched life and fragments of dreams is like. As small a shift as this would go a long way to making everything worthwhile.

My writing process would not be without personal benefits though as through my composition I learnt the joys and healing nature of the pen. Writing became my way to stand in the eye of the storm when everything else seemed to be sucked up into a tornado never to be seen again. Through this process I was reminded that life can go on after brain injury, it would just be up to me to make the most of it.

This seems to be a fitting place to stop, as I could go on rambling forever but would not want to be accused of circumlocution or using rather meaningless words just to pad my story. Avoiding a long-winded ending is almost as preferable as not living an exciting life. In the future, I can only hope that I can avoid the Chinese curse, "May you live in interesting times." I think I've had enough of that.

I hope that through my story you have been able to live my life vicariously through the ups and downs and catch a glimpse of a hidden world.

Although I used to think that my life was boring and there would be nothing really worth talking about, my adventure gave me more than enough material to fill several books. With such richness of experience, instead the challenge was to distil it down to just one. Writing this story was by turns challenging, wearisome and heartbreaking, yet also exciting, invigorating and contemplative. As you have persevered through to the end, I hope that you enjoyed the story of my journey and perhaps even found it fascinating, revealing and gripping.

As I close this chapter of my adventure, I would like to leave you with something to ponder. Next time you find yourself behind a ragged-looking traveller in the airport check-in line, a somewhat irate diner at the table next to you in a restaurant or opposite a smooth, suave lawyer in a boardroom, maybe tilting his head slightly to get a clearer view and find yourself increasingly exasperated, pause.

You never know, it could be me.

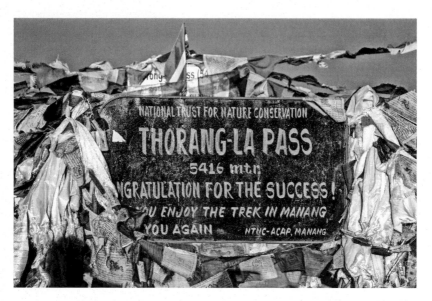

Photo copyright © Christopher Yeoh 2016 – Photo taken by the author Christopher Yeoh at Thorang-La Pass, Nepal. Shadow on the left is the author.

Epilogue

As editor of the Survivors' Stories series, I have been asked, and am very happy to accept the pleasurable task of writing an epilogue to this exceptionally brilliant and astonishingly honest account of life after severe brain injury. For the most part I shall draw heavily on the author's own words, in the main because they cannot be bettered; and on a few occasions I will allude to knowledge I have gained as an experienced neuropsychologist who has been, for forty years, involved in neuropsychological rehabilitation at both a practical level, as a researcher and as an author.

Readers will appreciate that the author of this volume has provided an account of life after brain injury that is unique in its depth of analysis and remarkably clever in its revelations as to what it is like to be brain injured and to progress from almost total dependence on others to the freedom of independence. Christopher has done this by, in his own words, "… trying to reframe [his] own little 'adventure' by changing [his] perspective so [he] could become the unbeatable hero in [his] own story." This changing of perspective is the backbone that runs throughout this book and is based upon changes that have taken place in the author as his recovery proceeds. It enables him to not only comment upon his circumstances and state of being at any one stage but to also analyse what he has gone through previously on his journey towards independence. It has meant moving initially from "a sad, blank and hopeless face propped up in a wheelchair in an empty corridor" to a "constructive member of society." Further, he describes his writing exercise as part of his recovery and his opportunity to widen understanding about traumatic brain injury: "[He] thought that in [his] re-writing of [himself] that maybe if [he] was lucky, who [he] wrote about and who [he] was … might merge together and become the truth. This writing would also be [his] chance to show the world that life after brain injury could still be full and fulfilling."

This positive outlook did not always come easily and there are times when the author has to fight against despair: at these times he felt as if he

"… was watching [his] own life without the chance to influence it … [his] emotions continued to flick between negative feelings so fast that it almost created a single mournful note." However, with remarkable fortitude the author overcomes such feelings, because he realises that it is "counterproductive to dwell on finger-pointing and blame" and he could not lead his life with a "millstone" of anger around his neck. This progression is perhaps best illustrated by the way the author changes his description of the initial mishap as an "accident" than a "crash," next to an "incident" and finally to an "adventure" from which can be drawn an uplifting story of a return to work and the fulfilment and pride which comes with that. He arrives at an eventual realisation that "sometimes the greatest adventures were those where the seemingly commonplace was made singularly extraordinary. It could be as simple as … making a solo trip to the corner shop or understanding when it was appropriate to cry."

The author continuously battles with negative feelings and comes out fighting with great spirit, seeing a way forward at each new set back as "inside [him] perfectionism, stubbornness and perseverance were vying with hopelessness, fear and apathy." The author's extraordinarily forceful personality is one of the reasons for such a positive outcome to his rehabilitation and the personal triumph that leads to his success in work and daily living – and of course to this powerful book. There are other attributes that have made the author's rehabilitation so successful despite the profound handicaps associated with traumatic brain injury. First of all, he is very intelligent – and he knows it – and this gives him great confidence. He was always successful at school and he admits to being a seeker of public acclaim. This was also seen in his sporting achievements where he pushed himself in physical adventures such as karate and triathlons. He freely admits to being a perfectionist, seeing beyond initial prejudices to a solid, honest assessment of rehabilitation ideas promulgated by any particular therapist, thus helping him to learn acceptance of his new self. He is always ready to take a second look. In fact, his progress is marked by a realisation that the "pursuit of perfectionism would not be so black and white anymore and life should be more balanced than that." The author is also capable of seeing the funny side of his many predicaments, none more so than when he sees beyond a therapist's stance to understand their intentions such as when he is followed supposedly secretly on a shopping expedition!

It is obvious that Christopher has a way with words: "[he] loved words and they loved [him] back"; "For [him], the story playing in [his] head painted through words was far more intriguing than physical success on the football field." And of course his chosen profession is law where ways with words are so vital. This particular personality trait was of particular use as during his recovery he read copious medical notes which "provided somewhere to start and a basis to seek further answers. The other way that [he] was able to relay the early days of recovery was to note 'interesting' events in a small notebook ... [which] was later to be a godsend for writing out [his] story."

It is unlikely that Christopher's intellectual achievements would have been so forthcoming after traumatic brain injury without considerable "cognitive reserve." The principle of cognitive reserve says that people with more education and high intelligence may show less impairment than those with poor education and low intelligence. Stern, in *Cognitive Reserve: Theory and Applications* (2007), suggests that individuals with high intelligence may process tasks in a more efficient way. He also reminds us that most clinicians are aware of the fact that any insult of the same severity can produce severe damage in one patient and minimal damage in another. This may also explain differences in recovery following non-progressive brain injury for, as Symonds in *Mental Disorder Following Head Injury* (1937) said in an often quoted remark, "it is not only the kind of head injury that matters but the kind of head."

According to Stern in *Cognitive Reserve: Theory and Applications* (2007), although there is no direct relationship between the degree of damage and the clinical manifestation of that damage, there are two separate models of cognitive reserve. One is a passive model which depends on the number of neurons possessed by an individual or the person's brain size, while the other is an active model whereby the brain uses its cognitive processing strategies or compensatory techniques to deal with the damage. Bigler in *Traumatic Brain Injury and Cognitive Reserve* (2007) believes that the passive model of cognitive reserve helps to explain not only the initial recovery from traumatic brain injury but also recovery across the lifespan.

At the end of his book Christopher suggests that he has even "overcome [his] adventure"; he does not have to pretend he is normal because he actually is. Further, successfully returning to work for him is recognition that brain injury survivors can still be constructive members of society and from now on he will "strive to be better rather than bitter." Through the journey recorded in his story, he has learnt not to look back in sadness at the past. Instead, he strives to face forwards as it is the future which matters.

A final point to make about Christopher's rehabilitation and the professional guidance he received from highly qualified therapists is that it has proved to be cost effective. He has returned to an extremely demanding job and is once again a valued member of society. As a lawyer he will be involved in matters that, if successfully resolved, will lead to a possible decrease in economic deprivation. He is active and pays his taxes. He is not a burden on either his family or society in general.

Obviously neuropsychological rehabilitation is time-consuming and expensive, especially in the early stages, but without it we would have a situation where affected families would have no escape from the constant attention that would be required to be given to the individual suffering from brain injury. Clinical rehabilitation can get individuals back to work in many cases and release families from possible unceasing care requirements. Its success can open up occupational opportunities; and it can lead in some cases to relational satisfaction that might otherwise be damaged because of untreated effects.

As Christopher's story shows, the consequences of brain injury should not be swept under the carpet; society must consider new ways of reducing health costs, especially with an ageing population. As the late Sir Keith Joseph once indicated, rehabilitation brings great dividends to society not only in terms of an increase in general health but also economically. The professionals working within neuropsychology are especially aware of this and are devising new ways of thinking and practising therapy, such as Community Based Rehabilitation, a system devised by the World Health Organisation. The aim being that people with disabilities, especially following an insult to the brain, must have equal opportunities to achieve good quality of life. Not only the affected individual but society will be better for it too.

Prof. Barbara A Wilson OBE, PhD, DSc,
CPsychol, FBPsS, FmedSC, AcSS
Clinical Neuropsychologist
January 2017

A little bit about the author

Christopher Yeoh is a holder of an LLB and LLM from the London School of Economics and practises securities law as a solicitor of England and Wales at a major global law firm.

After his adventure he now runs a multi-award winning food and travel blog at quieteating.com and is a featured photographer in the *Telegraph* and *Sunday Times* newspapers. His photos have also been featured in brochures by the luxury travel company, Audley Travel.

As an action man, he was previously an avid triathlete and a national award-winning karateka. Now he prefers a slower pace of life by writing and irritating people with his camera.

Life after brain injury is not something less – just something different.

References

Bauby, J. (2008). *The Diving Bell and the Butterfly*. London: Harper Perennial.

Baum, L.F. (reprinted 2015). *The Wonderful Wizard of Oz*. Creative Space Independent Publishing Platform.

Bigler E.D. (2007). Traumatic Brain Injury and Cognitive Reserve. In Y. Stern (ed) *Cognitive Reserve: Theory and Applications*. New York: Taylor & Francis.

Calderwood, L. (2008). *Cracked: Recovering After Traumatic Brain Injury*. London: Jessica Kingsley.

Cracknell, J., Turner, B. (2013). *Touching Distance*. London: Arrow.

Doidge, N. (2008). *The Brain That Changes Itself: Stories of Personal Triumph from the Frontiers of Brain Science*. London: Penguin.

Kahneman, D. (2011). *Thinking Fast and Slow*. London: Penguin Books.

Kushner, H. (2002). *When Bad Things Happen To Good People*. London: Pan.

Lewis, C.S. (1952). *Mere Christianity*. London: Geoffrey Bles.

Marsh, H. (2014). *Do No Harm: Stories of Life, Death and Brain Surgery*. London: W&N.

McCrum, R. (2008). *My Year Off: Rediscovering Life After a Stroke*. London: Picador.

Symonds, G.P. (1937). Mental disorder following head injury. *Proceedings of the Royal Society of Medicine*, 30, 1081–1094.

Stern, Y. (ed) (2007). *Cognitive Reserve: Theory and Applications*. New York: Taylor & Francis.

Tolkien, J.R.R. (reprinted 2007). *The Lord of the Rings*. London: HarperCollins.

Truss, L. (2009). *Eats, Shoots and Leaves*. London: Fourth Estate.

Wearing, D. (2005). *Forever Today: A Memoir of Love and Amnesia*. London: Doubleday.

Wilson, B.A., Robertson, C., Mole, J. (2015). *Identity Unknown: How Acute Brain Disease Can Destroy Knowledge of Oneself and Others*. New York: Psychology Press.

Further reading

Ross, M. (2013). *Rebooting My Brain: How a Freak Aneurysm Reframed My Life.*
   Washington: Red Slice Press.
Sachs, O. (2011). *The Man Who Mistook His Wife for a Hat.* London: Picador.
Sachs, O. (2011). *In the Mind's Eye.* London: Picador.
Toral, F. (2012). *Brain Injury: Where Do We Go from Here?* London: Tracy Porter.
Wilson, B.A., Winegardner, J., Ashworth, F. (2013). *Life after Brain Injury:
   Survivors' Stories.* New York: Psychology Press.

Index

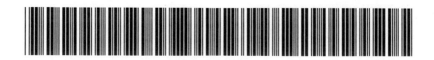